In the Midnight Hour,

Keep H.O.P.E. Alive!

Humility. Optimism. Participate. Embrace.

Patricia Henderson

In the Midnight Hour, Keep H.O.P.E. Alive!

ISBN (979-8-9858809-8-4)

Disclaimer: The following versions of the Bible may have been referenced: New International Version (NIV), King James Version (KJV), New Living Translation (NLT), English Standard Version (ESV), New King James (NKJV), New International Reader's Version (NIRV), Christian Standard Bible (CSB), Common English Bible (CEB), The Message (MSG).

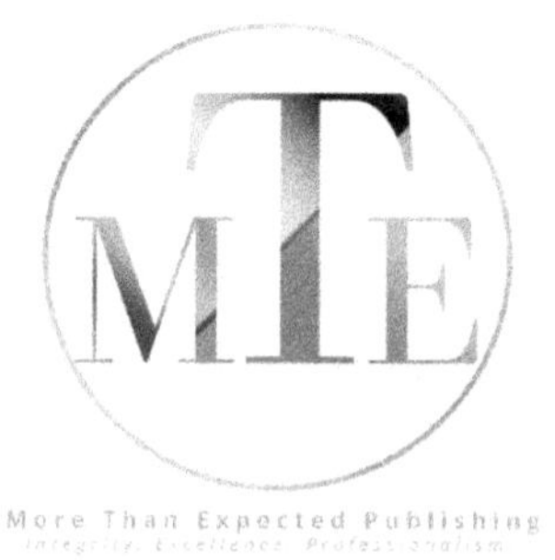

MTE Publishing
mtepublishing.com

Table of Contents

Dedication

This book is dedicated to everyone who has felt hopeless, I pray that you're encouraged to keep hope alive, no matter what!

Special Thanks & Acknowledgements

I give all honor and glory to my Lord and Savior, Jesus Christ for His grace, mercy, and wisdom.

To my husband, Charles, thank you for all your support and love. You have provided indescribable strength and encouragement throughout this project and our life journey.

To my children, Cedric [my daughter-in-love Janelle], Jacques and Devontrae, thank you for all your support and for being my inspiration to fight on.

To my grandchildren, Alicia, Ashlynn, and Christian, your smiles and love motivated Nana to keep writing when I wanted to give up.

To my mother-in-love, Momma-Mamie, you've done more for me than I ever expected. Thank you for being a second mom and friend to me. I love you, you accepted me from our first meeting.

To my brothers, Wendy, Calvin, Martine, Johnny, and Anthony, thank you for loving me completely and unconditionally.

Special thanks to Pastor Robert and First Lady Alicia Dowell, Pastor Linda Tucker [husband Billy Tucker], First Lady Shaun Bailey, and Elder Anthony and Joanne Aldridge for your love and support during one of the toughest seasons of my life.

Foreword

Pastor Linda M. Tucker

Years before I knew Patricia Henderson would be in my life, I walked beside my mother as she fought breast cancer. It was a path that was designated to increase my hope, in time. Heartbreakingly, as young girl, I witnessed the entirety of my mother's battle with cancer and her transition into eternity. I saw her suffer *hopelessly* at times. With technology not at its best, her doctors conducted uncertain procedures as they attempted to extend her life. However, their good intentions only crippled the quality of her life. At the age of 47, my mother's battle with cancer ended.

Our [Patrcia and I] coming together seemed random and to some of no consequence; however, I knew our meeting was divinely predestined. Almost from the very beginning, we knew we would be bound together by faith. We found ourselves drawn together through support and hope. As daughters whose mothers fatally battled breast cancer, we realized we had our battles to fight when we were diagnosed with breast cancer as well.

This book may not be one you choose without reason, but if you dare to look to God as your Source, pick it up, read it… You will get what you need. This literary work will remind you of your ultimate path within life. It will challenge you to see where you started and inspire you to believe that God has established your expected end. Although, hope is not microwaveable, it can be quickened. Hope can be built from a more substantial and unwavering foundation than you thought possible. Hope can change your perspective and ensure you live your best.

When life becomes *harder* for us, it is our faith in God and hope in Him that sustains us. We can win our battles as we look to Jesus, the "author and the finisher" of our faith. The words written herein offer hope. Patricia speaks the truth, layered with hope, marinated, and seasoned with love. She has lived through this from more than one angle and survived them all. Allow Patricia's journey to help you keep HOPE alive!

Pastor Linda M. Tucker, Th.D.

Introduction:
Her Story, My Story

My mother, Louise Brown was 75-years-old when she was diagnosed with stage III breast cancer in December 2008. I remember receiving a call late at night and my brother telling me mama was in the hospital. I could hear the fear in his voice as he tried to answer my questions. He gave the phone to my uncle, who tried to calm me down and reassure me that mama was ok. I asked him if I needed to make an emergency trip home, he quickly answered and said, "Let's wait until morning." Our call ended and I fell to my knees crying out to God to help my mother.

My mom was the pillar of strength in our family. She loved God and loved praying even more. I remember how she would have late night prayers with others over the phone. Every morning before she left for work, I saw her kneel by her bed to pray. She often encouraged my siblings and I to also pray and read the Word of God. She was a beautiful, happy, and faith-FULL woman. When faced with trials, her remedy for peace included prayer and Psalms 23. My mother was a warrior. She consistently worked, pressed forward and never complained about illness. She demonstrated how to be hopeful in seemingly hopeless situations.

During a sleepless night, I tossed and turned as worry set in concerning my mother. At daybreak, my phone rang. It was my Uncle. He informed me that I should prepare to make a trip home. He shared no update on my mother's condition but was insistent that I come home. My husband and I immediately began to search for flights to Florida. In the midst of preparation, our youngest son came to us complaining of a sore throat. Jumping into nurse mommy mode, I took his temperature, and sure enough, he had a fever. There was no doubt that I had to care for my son before traveling to Florida.

We scheduled an appointment at the clinic where I worked as a registered nurse. While the doctor was in the middle of his examination, my phone rang. I sprung up with anxiousness to quickly answer. The man on the other line spoke with a thick foreign accent. He introduced himself as Dr. Solar and told me that he was the doctor in charge of my mother's care. He reported that she had a large mass on her right breast; however, more in depth tests needed to be done.

I remember asking the doctor's opinion on whether or not I should make the trip to Florida… He replied, "Yes."

As I stood in the hallway of the clinic, my knees buckled, and I slid down the wall. A nearby staff nurse gently took my hand and asked if I was OK. As tears flowed from my eyes, my response to her was "no". After I regained control of my faculties, I returned to the exam room with my son and husband. When the examination was complete, we headed straight to the airport.

After we arrived in Florida, our main destination was the hospital. As I walked into the unit, I saw many family members in the waiting area. My Uncle Joseph met me in the hallway, and we embraced. He led me to the nurse so that she could brief me on what was happening with my mom. She guided me into a small private room and gave an update on my mother's health condition. Then I shared the information to my family before I entered my mother's room.

My mother was lying in the hospital bed with such a peaceful look on her face. She was hooked up to monitors and other machines. We were in the room alone. I asked her how she was doing, and I conducted a visual examination.

I saw the condition of her right breast. I had to ask her how long had she known about this? Her answer shook me to the core. She said, "It's been there for a while, and I didn't want to worry you or anyone else." At that moment, I felt as though I failed my mother. How could I miss this? How could I devote my life teaching others to perform preventive checks on themselves and forget about my own mother? A plethora of emotions consumed me in that moment, but I knew I had to shift my focus and be present for my mother.

A few days later after numerous tests, the diagnosis was stage III breast cancer. As I watched my mother walk through this valley, she demonstrated so much hope and positivity. Her strength amazed me as she went through chemotherapy, surgeries, and radiation. She held fast to her confession that "God was still in control". Her faith in God grew stronger during her journey and she graciously shared it with me at every opportunity.

After nearly a three-year battle, on June 28, 2011, mom passed. I spent the last five days of my mother's life at her bedside. The time we spent together was beautiful. Before her last breath escaped her lips, we both recited a sweet and simple "I love you." She left me with a smile that will forever be etched in my heart.

My mother's illness summoned me to my purpose. I immediately became a healthcare advocate stressing the importance of preventive care and self-breast exams. I made it my personal mission to share her story and educate others, especially those in my family. Losing my mom was a midnight hour for me and I often had to keep hope alive while experiencing the uncertainties of life without her. Naturally, I wondered what my chances were of being diagnosed with breast cancer.

Unfortunately, on April 28, 2017, mom's story became my story—it came for me, and I went after it, with my strength, mom's strength and most importantly, God's supernatural strength.

I've had an opportunity to meet many women over the years and sharing our stories is what connects us. I taught the women's group at my church on the topic of *Keep Hope Alive*. As I ministered to the ladies, I shared my breast cancer journey and how I was compelled to do just that. Being moved by the story, one of the ladies made it her business to personally encourage me. She said, "People need to know how you did it". In response to that encouragement, I decided to share H.O.P.E. and how remaining **humble** and **optimistic**, while **participating** in the plan, helped me to **embrace** my journey, face my fears, and walk in faith.

Thanks to my midnight hour [turned season], I am a better version of myself than I was prior to my diagnosis and after I beat cancer.

Chapter 1

Humility... Get Over Yourself [I did]

Life happens to each of us, no matter what. At some point in our lives, we will encounter a battle with hopelessness. Life is fragile and nothing is guaranteed. One phone call, one incident, or one moment in time can change our lives *forever*. On April 28, 2017, I received a phone call from my doctor's office requesting an appointment to review my radiology report. While in transit to the office, I became paralyzed with fear and anxiety. Suddenly, the sunny day became dark and gloomy.

A month prior, an annual mammogram procedure was scheduled in March. This is the time of year, when Spring cleaning begins, and winter items are tucked away. This particular year, the mammogram suite had been recently renovated. I was amazed at how modernized the area appeared. Several compliments were given to the staff on the renovated space. While filling out the paperwork, I nervously waited for the technician to call my name. I sat in the waiting area alone for what felt like hours but was actually only a few minutes. The technician finally called my name and escorted me to the dressing room to put on one of their gowns. While changing, I noticed signs that displayed information about breast cancer awareness posted on the walls. I tried my best to remain positive, but I couldn't help feeling anxious as I waited. I couldn't stop myself from thinking about mama's journey and her ultimate fate…

After a while, there was a knock at the door. The technician on the other side asked if I was ready; then she led me into the exam room. The procedure was explained and then performed. It included capturing several images of the area of concern. At the conclusion of the exam, the nurse informed me that the results would be sent through the mail. Feeling accomplished, I left the office and returned to work.

A few weeks later, I received a letter from the hospital containing my results. I opened the letter and expected to read "normal results, repeat in one year". However, the letter stated a repeat mammogram was necessary and needed to be scheduled. "Noooo!" I said, as my hands immediately went up in the air tossing the letter up with them. My husband was in the room with me. My reaction caused him to wonder what was going on. He told me not to think negatively and to schedule the appointment. The appointment was scheduled Tuesday, April 4, 2017.

At the follow up appointment, I was nervous and confused about the reasons for the repeat exam. The technician greeted me, and we started the mammogram. During the exam, more images were taken of the left breast than of the right breast. After the imaging was completed, I waited in the exam room. The technician returned and had to repeat a few more images. Although I was fearful and anxious, I remained calm and began to pray. This time the technician returned with the radiologist and informed me that there were some changes in my breast from the previous year. So, he recommended a biopsy as the next step. He told me what to expect and scheduled it right away. I selected a date, and the appointment was scheduled before I left the office that day.

I called my husband to inform him that I needed to have a biopsy done and scheduled it for April 17, 2017. I needed him to be with me. As I walked back to work, the sun shone bright and felt so warm to my skin. Surprisingly, I felt so calm in that moment. I returned to work and finished my day. After work, Charles and I briefly discussed my appointment. We didn't focus too much on it because it was our youngest son's birthday... We wanted the day to be all about him!

As the days passed, I remained productive at work and completed chores around the house. During this time, I was promoted to Chief Nurse of Ambulatory Care and traveled a few days a week to job sites which required overnight stays at a hotel. One night as I read my nightly devotional, the word valley came to mind. I wrote the word down in my notebook and searched the definition on Google. Valley, defined as a "low area of land between hills or mountains, typically with a river or stream flowing through it." As I pondered the definition and viewed several images associated with the word, tears flowed down my face. I began to praise God as I understood that even in the valley, God is still with me.

My daily routine consisted of spending time in prayer and reading the Word of God morning and evening. When I missed those alone times with God, I quickly noticed a difference in my day. As I reflected over my journey, God downloaded bits of information to prepare me for what was to come. The ever so soft voice was leading and guiding me through one of the darkest times in my life. I am forever grateful that I was able to perceive it.

The appointment day for the biopsy finally arrived. Charles and I woke up bright and early to prepare for what awaited us. I followed my routine of devotion and prayer while we drove to the hospital. We arrived at the suite area, checked in, and were greeted by the technician who performed my mammogram. I sat patiently waiting for my name to be called. After being called to the back, and then escorted to the dressing room, I was again taken to an exam room to be met by the radiologist.

Upon entry into the room, the radiologist and technician both greeted me and reassured me in the same instance. They then proceeded to explain the procedure and asked for my signed consent to continue with the process. During the preparation, I was in an extremely uncomfortable position. They tried their best to make me as comfortable as possible by adjusting the bed, but it just wasn't good enough.

As I lay there, I felt myself become anxious. I did my best to focus and remain calm enough to get through the procedure. At the start of it, I felt intense pain in my left breast, although the area of my breast was numb. The Technician did a well check and asked if I was alright. I replied, "No, I feel pain." The radiologist seemed surprised at my response. He applied a little more of the local anesthesia to numb the area and continued. He finished and reported that everything went well. He explained that the results would take about 10-14 days as specimens were processed in San Antonio, TX. He assured me that I would be contacted as soon as the results were in. The radiologist left the room while the technician applied bandages to the biopsy site, then I was escorted to the dressing room to recover my clothing, discharged, and released.

Charles and I walked to the car and recapped the conversations. To ensure there were no complications he instructed that I rest for the next few days. Since it was about lunch time, Charles and I ordered food to take back to the house. After lunch, the exhaustion of the day wore me down and I decided to take a nap. After a few hours of sleep, I was awakened by a soft voice calling my name. It was Charles, he had come into the bedroom to check on me. The pain from the procedure was much more intense than what I anticipated, so I continued to rest throughout the evening.

The next morning, I felt better, but still remained a little sore. Charles and I decided that it would probably be beneficial if I took another day off to recover. I contacted my supervisor to inform her I needed another day off. By day three, I noticed burning and itching near the site under the bandages. The area was monitored for a few more days; however, the pain became more intense. Once the tape came off, I realized because of my sensitive skin I was having a reaction to the tape. I made an appointment with my primary care provider (PCP) to assess the area and prescribe medication. After about a week the process of healing began. I currently bear a scar to this day that reminds me of that journey and encourages me to keep hope alive.

Chapter 2

Optimism is Absolutely Necessary

A week passed and I still hadn't received any correspondence from the doctor. Life continued, and I tried not to give much thought to my pending results.

On a sunny Friday afternoon, while I sat in my office I received a text from a nurse, who was also a friend of mine; she worked at my doctor's office. She asked if I was working in a specific area that day but didn't reveal why she wanted to know. I responded, "No…" and waited for her response, but she didn't say anything.

A little while later, the phone rang. It was the clinic. Nervously, I answered the phone. The woman on the other end politely asked to speak with Patricia Henderson. "I'm Patricia, I replied." She introduced herself and told me she was calling from the X-ray department. She explained that the doctor needed me to come in as soon as possible to discuss the results of the exam.

Before I left work, I sat at my desk for a few minutes feeling nervous and anxious. I fumbled around as I attempted to turn off my computer and put away my things. My supervisor was out of the office at the time, and she was the only one that knew of my impending health situation. In her absence, I needed to inform the chief nurse on duty. I knocked on her door, she waved for me to come in. I entered the office and closed the door behind me. She told me to have a seat, but I was so nervous, I remained standing and paced back and forth. I explained my situation and told her that I needed to leave for the day. She quickly responded saying, "Yes, go!" as she stood from her desk to embrace me.

I went back to my office and quickly gathered my belongings and headed to the car. The parking area was a little distance from the hospital campus. On a normal day, I took the shuttle to the parking area, but this day, I walked the full distance. I walked as fast as I could to get to my car. I tried calling my husband, but he did not answer the phone. I called his office, and he was not in. I left a message for him to call me as soon as possible. When I finally made it to the car, my heart was pounding, my hands were sweating, and the nervous feeling lingered in the pit of my stomach. As I prepared to leave the parking area, my phone rang. It was

Charles. I informed him about the call; I asked him to meet me at the clinic.

In my travels from Oklahoma City to Fort Sill, I played my favorite gospel praise music in an attempt to calm my nerves. I knew I had to stay calm to safely drive to the clinic. As I listened to the music, I began to pray loudly and boldly declare scriptures of healing. As I prayed and praised, the feeling of worship began to wash over me, and tears began to flow. I honestly don't remember most of the drive, but I do remember feeling a sense of peace and safety.

Upon arrival, I whipped into the first available parking space I could find. I was about to call Charles, when all of a sudden, I looked to my left and there he was in the parking space right next to me. I grabbed my purse and exited the car. Charles and I walked hand in hand as we made our way towards the clinic. When we entered, I saw several familiar faces (past coworkers and personnel staff). They waived hello as we walked by. I was formerly employed at this particular clinic for many years and am well known throughout the facility.

We made it to the X-ray department. I went to the counter, gave the clerk my name, and was directed inside. She picked up the phone and called someone and informed them that I had arrived. She instructed me to have a seat, and someone would be with me shortly.

Charles and I sat patiently in the waiting room. We watched as several patients came in and out of their scheduled appointment. As I sat and waited for the doctor, my heart pounded hard against the walls of my chest making it difficult to breathe. It felt as though I was having a panic attack. I grabbed Charles' hand and focused on controlling my breathing. This feeling lasted only a moment but felt like an eternity. My body was on its way back to a calm state when I looked out of the window facing the hallway and saw my PCP and a case manager walk around the corner. My heart sank!

From my clinical employment experience, I was familiar with protocol when it came to informing patients of abnormalities in test results concerning Women's Health. The team entered and walked to the back. I pointed out the identities of the two women on the team to Charles and confirmed that this was not a good situation.

As I waited, my legs shook uncontrollably. I tried my best to remain positive. In the background I heard, "Mrs. Henderson," in a feminine tone. I looked back and it was the technician who conducted the mammogram and biopsy. Charles and I stood up to meet her. She greeted us both as we walked towards the suite. As we got closer to the designated area, I saw Mrs. Bowman, my PCP, and Mrs. Adams, case manager. The closer I got to the door, the louder my ears rang from the intense beating of my heart.

When I entered the exam room, I screamed and cried. Charles along with the technician helped me to the chair. Mrs. Bowman said, "Do you already know the results?" Charles held me tightly in his arms as I continued to cry. The technician wiped my face and held my hand. She was attentive and caring; her acts of kindness meant so much to me. I don't remember her name, but her compassion will be forever held close to heart.

Charles was very patient with me and politely instructed everyone else to do the same. He continued to console me and would gently remind me to calm down. I tried as best as I could to calm down. Often, when I am upset or nervous, I hold my hands together and place them under my chin. I used this calming technique while silently repeating to myself that everything is going to be fine.

Mrs. Bowman asked, "Do you know the results?" I responded, "No, I do not." The moment I entered the room, so many memories of my mom surfaced; not to mention the anticipation of the fate that awaited me.

The feeling in that instance caused the tears to flow uncontrollably. Mrs. Bowman reported the biopsy results as a diagnosis of Ductal Carcinoma in Situ (DCIS). Those words sent shock waves through my body. I was emotionally overwhelmed. The case manager chimed in, "No cancer is good but this one is not a bad one." I undoubtedly agreed to the statement that n*o cancer is good*. Every word spoken afterward was muffled.

Talk about surgeons and oncologists was tossed around. I wasn't ready to discuss this all at once. I needed some time to process and research. I responded, "Give me the weekend to think about this... I don't know any providers." Mrs. Bowman and Mrs. Adams agreed to revisit the conversation at a later date. Mrs. Adams gave me her business card as the point of contact when I was ready. They reassured me that I was going to be alright and that this was not a death sentence. As I listened to the words that so easily belted out of their mouths, I reflected on times when I had to give that same speech to patients in my care—It hits much *differently* when a cancer diagnosis is yours!

The appointment ended and it felt as though time had stopped and I was unsure of what would be next. I felt numb. What just happened? Charles and I embraced one another as we walked to the car in silence. When we got closer to the car, we noticed I had a flat tire. As I glanced over the tire, all I could say was, *thank you Lord!* Charles said, "Let's leave in the truck and we will come back later to pick up the car."

As we drove home, I thought of individuals that may be able to help me through this process. I really needed my mom, but unfortunately, she was no longer with us. Even though I could not pick up a physical phone to talk with mom, I felt her spirit so close to me. I thought of the next best person to call, Elder Tucker. She is like a mother figure to me and a breast cancer survivor. I knew her calming voice and inspiring story would be just what I needed to help soothe my nerves.

We arrived home and sat quietly in the living room for a few minutes. I called Elder Tucker and put the call on speaker. She answered the phone and said "Hello, Minister Henderson." I responded "hello," I asked, "are you busy?" She replied, "Billie and I were talking... What do you need?" Warm tears flowed down my face and my voice trembled, I said "I was diagnosed with breast cancer." She said, "Oh, no Minister Henderson." I continued to tell her what the doctors said. Then she asked, "Do you want to live?" I replied "Yes." She said, "Now we can continue." She began to share her journey with me along with the names of the doctors she used... Her words were so encouraging. She took a few minutes to talk with Charles and encouraged him also. Before our call ended, she said a prayer and promised to keep in touch. I felt so much better after our talk. Speaking with Elder Tucker reminded me of who I was and *whose* I was on this journey.

When I heard the diagnosis of cancer, I wondered... Why me? What did I do wrong? As a registered nurse, I educated others on the importance of monthly self-breast exams, annual mammograms, and physicals with their provider. I was very diligent with my health regimen, especially after losing mama. So, the shock of my diagnosis seemed to be more than I could bear. Fortunately, I realized that the mammogram saved my life.

After cancer claimed the life of my beloved mom and other family members, I shared preventive measures that would potentially save their lives. Ask yourself, when was the last time you visited your doctor for your annual preventive screening? I had no symptoms and felt no lumps. Consequently, within a year there was a change in my mammogram, and it was cancer. I encourage you to take control of your health. Face your fears, stop now and schedule your mammogram; temporary discomfort of a screening is far better than not knowing… Prevention is key.

I read a proverb that says, "It's easier to stop something from happening, in the first place, then to repair the damage after it's done."

According to the American Cancer Society, you can help reduce your risk of cancer by making healthy choices like eating right, staying active and not smoking. They also highly recommend annual cancer screenings.

Facing My Cancerous Reality

Charles and I went out to dinner for a mental break. We discussed how we'd share the news with our children and families. Our youngest son and nephew were in the final semester of their sophomore year of college. They had about two weeks before their semester final exams. We decided that we would not break the news to our boys because of the impact it could have on their academic performance. Our eldest son and family lived in Raleigh, NC at the time. I know my boys love and care for me dearly and I wanted them to know, but we had to find the perfect time to tell them. I reflected on the loss of my mother and how it impacted them when we lost her to cancer and how much they worried about me during that time. We agreed that we would tell our boys after more information was received. However, we decided to tell our oldest son much sooner and asked him not to tell his brothers.

We finished dinner and returned to the clinic to fix the flat tire. I sat in the truck watching Charles and my thoughts were all over the place. Charles quickly changed the tire and walked to my side of the truck. I let the window down and he spoke these very words to me, "As I changed the tire, the Lord said to me,' just as easy as it was for you to change the tire, this process will be just that easy.'" I replied, "Amen!" He reminded me of a previous challenge we experienced when we had a flat tire on this car. He had to call a tow truck to change the flat tire. We both smiled at each other and knew that despite what we were facing God was, is, and will always be in charge. We drove separately back to our home and prepared to spend a quiet evening together.

After a long hot shower, I walked into the bedroom and told Charles I felt lost and hopeless. He reassured me that everything was going to be alright. I was in a place I had never been before. I was constantly helping others in this situation, but cancer knocked on my door and I didn't know how to answer. I was afraid… Oh how quickly life changes! I started my day with such joy and determination as I set out to check off some of the many tasks; However, the nights led me to wonder if I would live or die.

Charles was a great listener. He allowed me to share my feelings, but he would not allow me to continue to rehearse the problem. I know the diagnosis was just as devastating to him as it was to me, but he remained positive and helped me to do the same.

During this journey, I quickly learned I had to humble myself and allow others to help me. As a woman with many roles, wife, mother, nana, minister, nurse, and leader, it is common to care and think of others first. This time, I was the one that needed the care. I was in a very unfamiliar place, and I needed help. My life changed overnight. I had the responsibility to change with it because if I did nothing, fear and hopelessness would creep in and overtake me. Although difficult, I understood the power of my thoughts and actions would impact my battle plan. I learned that faith coupled with optimism are key strategies for winning the first war that happens in the mind. My first order of business was to solicit prayers, from my family and friends, to cover my mind. I didn't want my thoughts to spiral. I needed to stand firm in my faith to beat this thing! I had to finish what mama started.

The day I received the diagnosis of breast cancer was unforgettable. The very thought that this disease could possibly take me from my family was unbearable. I made the decision to humble myself, trust God, trust the doctors and allow my family and friends to help me every step of my uphill journey.

As a registered nurse, I had to shift roles from caregiver to patient. My knowledge and experience of caring for patients with cancer, could have hindered my journey. Although I knew enough about the disease from mom's experience and my 25- plus years of healthcare experience; there was no room for arrogance or ego. I had to listen. There were so many things going through my mind. Then I finally made the decision to humble myself and surrender this battle to God's perfect will. I felt more at peace, and I walked in the steps that God ordered. This is how I kept hope alive. This is not something that happened over night. This was and is a process I continuously practice today.

Honestly, trusting God in the process was not the challenge but trusting others was. I experienced hurt and disappointment from people I thought were loving and loyal. This was another war, learning to be vulnerable. Many people may believe that I am antisocial, withdrawn, or too private. None of those things are true. However, I am cautious about who I allow in my space and in my inner circle.

While in the fight of my life, I had to protect my inner circle to stay alive. Everyone had an opinion of what should or should not be done, but the ultimate decision was mine and mine alone. I had to keep my strength for the race I was called to run. I understood before any race, the runner must be well rested and prepared to face the challenges ahead. Practicing humility allowed me to R.E.S.T. — **recognize** I need help; **express** how I feel; **seek** feedback/help from others and **treasure** moments. This is how hope began to arise in my midnight hours (that would come sporadically at any given time). I also call these midnight moments.

Chapter 3

Overcoming Obstacles

Early Saturday morning, I awoke feeling refreshed. To start our day, Charles and I ate a well-balanced breakfast. Our car needed a new tire, so Charles went to purchase a new one. While he was out, I sat alone with my thoughts. I relaxed on the sofa and began my morning devotional time with God. However, I still felt a bit numb from the news. So, I prayed and asked God to give me wisdom, strength, and healing for what was to come. I started to cry, I heard a soft voice say, "This is for your family, and you will be alright." Immediately, I resolved within myself that I had to go through this to stop this disease from crossing over to other generations in our family; this was a divine assignment. I am a strong believer in the power of prayer, and I know God speaks to us if we have an ear to hear.

I walked around my living room, praising God in that moment; I truly believed I'd be OK. I recorded that experience in my journal for future reference. I completed some housework that day and felt better and stronger as the day went on. I texted a former colleague and PCP for advice on local doctors to use for my care. She informed me she was out of town and would contact me upon her return.

The following day, we went to church. We decided to share the news with our pastors and met with them briefly before service. As we stood in the pastor's office, my husband shared the news that I had breast cancer. They gave us a surprised, yet, concerned look and asked questions. We answered what we could since it was too early in the process. They prayed with us and then we went into service and had an awesome time. Even with the unfavorable diagnosis I had recently received, I was determined to give God praise. While in church, I received a text from my previous PCP that read, "Are you able to talk right now?" I replied, "I am in church at the moment, can we schedule a time to speak a little later."

Charles and I returned home and had Sunday dinner. I called Dr. Schafer, my previous PCP. Our call started with reconnecting with each other. It had been about three years since we last communicated. After we caught up, I told her about my diagnosis and asked for recommendations regarding my care. She expressed her sorrowfulness in my struggle, then she educated me on advancements in treatment of DCIS. She also offered her consolation that I would be fine. She gave the name of a recommended surgeon and two names for oncologists.

After the call, I reflected on the times that I scheduled appointments to see Dr. Schafer concerning my left breast (from years past). At that time, she developed a treatment plan that included routine exams but concluded that my breasts were fibrous (lumpy/rope-like texture). However, the left was more fibrous than the right.

Dr. Schafer was an amazing doctor. She continued to listen and made me feel comfortable with any medical concerns I presented to her. I took down the names that she recommended. One of the names sounded very familiar. I discovered it was the same doctor responsible for Elder Tucker's care when she went through her battle with breast cancer.

Later that evening, Charles and I called our eldest son through FaceTime to share the news with him. We asked the whereabouts of his wife because we wanted them to support each other as we told them the news. At the time, we had two granddaughters and I could hear one of them in the background and the other one sat on her mother's lap. Charles told Cedric that I'd been diagnosed with breast cancer. Before we could say another word, Cedric let out a scream and began to cry. I had not expected that type of reaction from him. The look of disbelief on his face shattered my heart. I tried to stay strong and not let him see me cry as our granddaughter came over to comfort her dad. I watched as she asked him, "Dad what is wrong?" Her actions next touched my heart as she laid her head over the left side of his chest and comforted him. Charles held my hand, I shared what the doctor said, and assured them that I'd be fine. I noticed the look on his wife's face, and I asked if she was OK, but she didn't respond. I asked again and got no response.

My son said, "Mama, she's OK." We shared our decision not to tell his siblings yet and the reasons why. He agreed he would not say anything to them. I told him I would keep him updated after all of the follow up appointments. We ended our call with much sympathy and love. I sat on the sofa, phone in hand reflecting on the pain I felt in my heart for my child. I can only imagine the memories of his grandmother [my warrior] that flashed through his mind as I shared the news.

This was my deepest fear. For this reason, I wrestled with the idea to tell them. I wanted to hold my son in my arms and comfort him. At that moment, I wanted to protect him from the pain he experienced. I told Charles how I felt, and I remember him saying, "I love how you are still protecting us in the midst of what you are going through." I smiled at him, and we embraced each other. I prepared for my work week and went to bed.

At work on Monday, I sat in a morning huddle with the other chief nurses. I was completely unfocused. Terri, the chief nurse, observed the look on my face and out of concern she asked, "Are you OK?" I shook my head side-to-side to indicate that I wasn't. My eyes welled with tears but I quickly refocused so I would not cry. I made it through the morning report and quickly went to my office.

While I reviewed the calendar for the day, there was a knock at my door, it was my supervisor. She sat in the chair next to my desk and began to share about her time off. She asked, "Did you get your results?" Before I could answer, she said "I had been thinking about you all weekend." She shared that Terri texted her on Friday to tell her I was going to get my test results.

As she spoke, my eyes teared up again. I told her my results were positive for cancer. This time I couldn't hold back the tears. She replied, "I am so sorry Patricia." She asked me of my plans, I told her I did not know. She shared a story of her friend who was diagnosed with breast cancer. I asked her not to share with others since I had not told all my family yet. She agreed and we continued our conversation for a few more minutes. She left my office and I continued with my day.

Tuesday morning, additional appointments were set with Mrs. Adams. I gave her the name of the general surgeon I wanted to meet with, she took note of that to coordinate my appointments. After a few hours, Mrs. Adams gave me a return call to give me the solidified dates of the appointments. I was surprised at how quickly my appointment was scheduled. Mrs. Adams reminded me that she will be coordinating my care and if I needed anything to contact her directly.

I kept Charles informed of all appointments and conversations every step of the way. Arrangements were made with my supervisor concerning my appointments at the Lawton Outpatient Clinic in Lawton, OK. Which was quite the distance from my place of employment. At the end of my workday, I traveled to the hotel where I would stay for the night. I tried to conduct a normal routine, but the longer I sat in the room, the more my mind wandered about everything that I was going through. On the outside, I tried to remain calm and positive, but I was terrified. It seemed as if praying and crying was the norm. In the middle of my tears, my phone rang. Yes, it was Charles. I quickly cleared my throat to not give any indication that I was sad and crying. I believe he felt the need to call me at that very moment.

When the time came for my appointment with Dr. Hunter, Charles accompanied me. As I walked through the halls of the building, my mind could not process the fact that I was going to consult a doctor to discuss my options as a cancer patient. When we made it to the designated area, I checked in at the front desk. The clerk was very polite as she gave me what seemed to be a whole novel to complete.

As I completed the papers, I looked around the waiting area and saw people from all walks of life, waiting their turn to be seen by the doctor. I wondered why they were here and what thoughts were going through their minds. I completed the packet, returned it to the clerk, and made my way back to my seat. The more I waited, the more nervous I became. I had to do something quick to shift my thoughts. Of course, you guessed it, I turned to my devotional to help me fight this battle.

After what seemed like a wait for eternity, the nurse finally called my name. Charles and I followed her as she gave a pleasant greeting. She verified my identification by asking my full name and date of birth. After she completed the screening process, she calmly exited the room and stated that dreaded phrase, "The doctor will see you soon."

Dr. Hunter entered the room with a welcoming smile and sincere greetings. She reviewed my health history and asked more questions while examining the biopsy results. My heart raced as if I were running for my life. I was so afraid of what was happening my voice trembled with each response. Dr. Hunter recognized the fear in my tone. She stopped the questions for a moment and allowed me time to gather myself. Further assessment of my breast was needed so I "gowned up". During the manual exam, she asked, "Did you feel anything on your exams?" I replied, "No, I did not." As she continued to examine my breast, she scanned the report once again and said, "I don't feel anything either." It was determined that the next step was to schedule an MRI.

When the nurse entered the room again, I gave her the names of two oncologists that I wanted to handle my case, Dr. Garza, and Dr. Robin. She confirmed that they were both excellent doctors. I continued to discuss my options with Dr. Hunter. We discussed possibilities of surgery. One option was called a lumpectomy. However, the results of the MRI would determine if we needed to explore other options. I was provided information pamphlets on breast cancer while she shared information about reconstructive surgery and insurance payments. The nurse returned to the exam room with an appointment with Dr. Garza and they confirmed my appointment for an MRI.

Before leaving the room, Dr. Hunter wanted to know if we had any questions. I didn't know how to answer that because I had so many questions. I needed time to process all of it. Good thing the doctor gave the OK to call if I had any questions prior to my appointment. My calendar was getting booked with all the appointments I set. Truthfully, I was overwhelmed with everything. Even in the middle of this, I still had a difficult time wrapping my mind around the fact that *I had cancer.* Fear of the unknown caused so much anxiety that I could barely function.

Later that day, I received a call from the MRI clinic, confirming the appointment. The scheduler provided the instructions for the MRI procedure and directed me to contact my provider for calming medication, if needed. I recalled getting an MRI of my neck a few years prior. I had major difficulties remaining calm while inside of the imagining machine. So, I decided I needed some form of medication this time around. The medication was ordered, and I picked it up the next day.

While in wait mode, I decided to get educated about my diagnosis and treatment options. The options that best fit in my situation were lumpectomy or double mastectomy. What I really wanted was for this to be over and done with! Whatever option I chose, I wanted the outcome to be that I would never have to deal with cancer again. In the decision process, I was leaning more towards a double mastectomy. I shared my thoughts with Charles; he listened and replied with a sweet and soft-spoken tone, "I support whatever you decide, and I will be here with you through it all." I also read the literature on reconstructive surgery, but at that moment all I was concerned about was serving cancer an immediate eviction notice. I'd focus on the clean up after the fact.

Here we are, appointment day. To keep my life functioning as normally as possible, I kept my day-to-day schedules somewhat consistent. I went to work for a couple of hours before my appointment. Charles met me at the clinic. I never imagined I would be coming in for an appointment in this building. The clerks at the desk were very polite as I went through the check-in process. While I sat in the waiting area, I looked around at the other patients. They appeared much older than I was and some frail in health. As I waited, I thought about the times I accompanied my mother to her appointments. This was beginning to feel way too real; I picked up a magazine in an effort to distract my worrying.

The same routine was followed with every visit. When the nurse completed her mission, Dr. Garza entered the room. Her smile was so calming and radiant. She introduced herself and began the process of reviewing and diagnosis. She explained the disease in depth and informed me of the processes involved. She explained that the most ideal treatment for DCIS would be the lumpectomy. A double mastectomy was far too aggressive for this type of cancer. She further explained that she was the attending physician who would take over after the outcome of the surgery and results had been determined. More questions about my family history were investigated. Most questions I could not answer because I had no clue. In order to get a better understanding of what may be, Dr. Garza recommended genetic testing. Insurance options were researched concerning the cost and coverage of the screening. In most instances, genetic testing is covered, depending upon the individual's risk factors.

Towards the end of the visit, Dr. Garza completed an examination and answered all of our questions. A visit with the social worker was recommended as she assisted in navigating my appointments.

We briefly met with the social worker, and she shared information on additional services offered at the Cancer Center of Southwest Oklahoma. These services included counseling and support groups. I received a lot of pamphlets and points of contact; in case I had any questions. As we walked out to our cars, I was attempting to process what happened. I returned to work and tried to focus on the tasks at hand, but it was very difficult to concentrate. Later that evening, my husband and I talked briefly as we reflected on the visit with Dr. Garza. I was surprised at how much I did not know about my extended family. There was hearsay about the cause of death of my maternal grandmother as well as some other family members. However, I was unaware of any details pertaining to medical conditions surrounding their deaths. I later reached out to some family members to get a little more information on their medical history while keeping my situation under wraps.

A few days later, we arrived at the clinic for the MRI appointment. I was amazed at how nice the clinic looked. The decorations and colors were so soothing that it gave the clinic a feel of calm and relaxation. Prior to my arrival, I had taken the medication prescribed to help me relax during the MRI. Shortly after check-in, the technician called my name. This time Charles was unable to accompany me back. This made me a little more nervous than I was already. I was taken to a maze of rooms. One room to change, another room to have an IV placed, and ultimately the MRI room. In the past, to get over the fear of this procedure, I would close my eyes to dismiss the focus of the machine. This time was a little different. Upon entering the room, the machine was front and center. To my surprise, it was an open MRI. The previous ones didn't have a large opening, and they triggered my claustrophobia.

The tech supplied me with headphones to listen to my favorite music to drown out the sound of the machine. Additionally, instead of lying on my back, I was instructed to lie on my stomach. The music played as the table began to move toward the machine. I closed my eyes and prayed. The music was calming and took my focus off the noise from the machine. After a few minutes the technician returned to the room and said, "You're all done."

She took me to another room, removed the IV and I returned to the dressing room. When I came out, Charles was right there waiting for me. I was a little dizzy from the medication, so to make sure I was OK, I went home and rested for the remainder of the day.

Two days later, I had a follow up appointment with Dr. Hunter. She informed us of the results from the MRI… The good news was the MRI showed results similar to that of the biopsy. She was confident that we found the cancer early and it was contained in the ducts. Now, it was time to discuss surgical options.

After reading all the material, talking with both doctors, and praying, I made the decision to have the lumpectomy. A lumpectomy is a surgical procedure that removes cancerous breast tissue along a surgical margin, which is the rim of connecting normal tissue. This procedure preserves the healthy portions and sensations of the breast. Dr. Hunter explained what we should expect during surgery and recovery. She also informed us that if the surgical margin was not clear, it would require more surgery. We scheduled the surgery for the following week. I felt good about our visit and my decision.

Charles and I had decided to go to our boy's track meeting in Shawnee, OK for the weekend. All of the things happening with me was during National Nurses Week, and I needed to be at work for the award ceremony. I attended the ceremony with the other chiefs and presented the awards to my staff. We had a great time and one of the nurses was surprised she received the award. My team had contacted her family and informed them she was receiving an award. Her family surprised her at the event. When we called her name, their cheers brought tears to her eyes.

After the celebration, I shared with my supervisor how my appointment went and the decision I made for surgery. The look on her face made me feel as though I made the wrong choice. I struggled the rest of the day, wondering if I made the right decision. That one reaction brought back the doubt and fear that I thought had subsided.

My workday was complete and all I could think about was getting food and seeing our boys. When Charles and I connected again, I told him about my day. I shared the fun had by all at the award ceremony and also the response given by my supervisor after I revealed my decision. He encouraged me not to worry and to be secure with the choice that I made. We arrived at our hotel, unpacked, and went to dinner. After dinner we walked around the hotel and enjoyed the sites before heading back to our room.

As I prepared for bed, I had such a feeling of fear and doubt that I did not sleep well at all that night. My thoughts were racing, I tossed and turned all throughout the night. I awoke early the next morning, grabbed my iPad, and went into the bathroom so as not to wake Charles. I was scared and did not know what to do. I sat on the floor in the bathroom and prayed "Lord, I need You!" Tears flowed from my eyes as I asked God to give me a sign on how to handle what I was facing. I opened my iPad to the Bible App and the scripture for the day was 2 Corinthians 12:9, *My grace is sufficient for you, for my power is made perfect in weakness.* I read the scripture over and over until it settled in my spirit. As tears flowed down my face, I praised God. I knew that His Word would be the lamp unto my feet and the light unto my path, particularly on this journey. As I continued to sit on the floor, I noticed the nervous feeling subsided. I continued to praise, without getting too loud because Charles was asleep. That was my power hour and I shifted divinely — from fear to faith!

I collected myself and prepared for my morning routine. I got into the shower. As the water hit the base of the tub, I recalled speaking at my local church during a

Women's Conference. The women were encouraged to give $70; the number 70 means spiritual perfection.

God reminded me of the seed I had sown, at that time, and how that seed perfected my faith in this season. I finished my shower and wrote the following declaration in my journal:

> *Seventy equals spiritual perfection. Father God, You told me after all of this is over, it will be in the seventh month, and it will be completed. My new beginning will start. Father, I trust You. You have not failed me yet and You will not fail me. Lord, I thank You!*

I sat at the desk reflecting on what I wrote and praised God for His faithfulness. We made it to the track meet. I was so happy to see our boys. As they embraced me with a strong hug, it was hard to keep my condition a secret. I tried hard to mask my feelings and not let my facial expressions tell the story that something was wrong. The track meet began, and the crowd cheered. As I watched them run their races, I was so proud of them and wanted to protect them from anything that could harm them, including the information that I had to share.

In between the races we caught up through casual conversations. Their faces lit up as they talked about school and other interests. I saw their smiles and heard such joy in their voices. As we went throughout our day, being around them became easier. After we left the meet, we had dinner and shared life, laughter, and love as we talked about the ups and downs.

Final exam week was approaching for our sons, after their test they would be home. I thought, "In just a few more days, I can share my diagnosis and treatment strategy with them." We said our goodbyes and prepared for our trip home.

It was a quiet drive back to Lawton, OK. I enjoyed our time together but felt sad wondering how the news would impact our boys. As I gazed at the sunset, I took the opportunity to thank God for His many blessings. Later that evening, I called my brothers to share the news with them. I have five brothers and we are very close. I knew this news would be hard for them and would bring up memories of our momma's battle with breast cancer.

Since our mother's death, my brothers have looked up to me and depended on me as they did with our mom. At times, it was challenging but other times it was rewarding. Our bond as siblings grew closer after mom passed. We all realized that we must remain in unity to keep her legacy alive. I was able to contact four of my brothers that night. With each call I made, the news of my illness became harder to repeat, and saying these three words, "I have cancer" deeply saddened me. Also, not knowing how everyone would react weighed heavily upon my heart.

The silent pauses from each one of them caused more tears and emotions of uncertainty. Nevertheless, it seemed as though I was more concerned with consoling everyone else after I shared my news. This was crazy when I was the one with the cancer diagnosis. I'd encourage them as I encouraged myself by saying things like, "I'll be alright," "I'm strong and I will get through this," "Don't worry God's in control." Although deep down, I wasn't sure if I believed any of that for myself.

A few days passed and it was almost time for surgery. I met with my staff to share the news with them to discuss coverage while I was on leave. Our huddle started with the usual roll call then we briefed on upcoming tasks for the days ahead. My voice trembled as I shared my condition with the staff. When the words "I have cancer" fell from my lips the call went silent. One by one each spoke up and I could hear the concern in their voices. Darlene, one of the nurse managers, offered encouragement in her own way and said, "Patricia, I am sorry to hear this but if anyone can beat this, it is you!" At that moment, I felt empowered. Hearing her say those words was so touching. I realized that the strength and faith she saw in me, I had to recognize in myself. After a few more words of encouragement, tears, and laughter, we ended our call and continued our workday.

Before my next meeting, I went to the cafeteria to get a cup of coffee. I saw one of my staff members and we greeted each other and talked while we waited in line. I shared with her that I would be out for a few days because of my health situation. I uttered those dreaded words once again, "I have breast cancer." She stopped in her tracks and suggested that we go to my office. We purchased our items quickly and scurried to my office. We further discussed that I was set for surgery the following day and we also discussed the chosen treatment option.

Because of the nature of her career as an advanced practice registered nurse, she was prompted to ask questions and offer her expertise on what to expect in surgery and how to care for myself afterwards as far as my diet to help promote healing. Over the years, our relationship grew from cordial colleagues to good friends. What she did next surprised me but was much needed and appreciated. She held my hands and prayed for me. Her prayers were so powerful and anointed.

As she prayed, tears flowed down my face, and she embraced me with a hug. Her touch was what I needed at that very moment. She was one of the angels, God placed in my path to help keep hope alive. Throughout my journey, she would send me scriptures and prayers through texts. The acts of kindness that she displayed were truly heart felt, sincere, and pure. To this very day, we continue as sisters in Christ to uplift and encourage one another.

The night before surgery, our youngest son came home from college. He finished out the semester and was home for a few weeks. I was so unsure as to how he would react to the cancer news. We allowed time for him to unpack and settle in before we requested to speak with him. Charles called him into the living room where I sat on the sofa and Jacques stood just within my reach. I explained the situation to him from start to finish. I started with the results of the mammogram and biopsy and ended with the diagnosis of DCIS breast cancer and surgery [the following day].

He sat next to me with a look of shock and fear on his face. I told him that I waited to tell him because I wanted him to remain focused on his studies to successfully close out the semester. We embraced each other and he looked me in my eyes and said, "You are such a strong woman, and you will show your strength as you walk through this." We moved on to more uplifting conversations. I was surprised at how well he handled the news. I expected him to be the one to really react irrationally, instead it was my older son that had the hardest time dealing with the news.

I only had two more people left to tell, my nephew and another brother. There were several attempts to call my brother, but each time there was no answer. My nephew still had two more exams to take before he could be able to come home. I anticipated and tried to imagine what their reactions would be, but I tried not to worry too much about that.

Since my surgery was scheduled for the following day, I continued to prepare.

The next day, we reported to the hospital by 6 a.m. I woke up early to prepare my mind since most of the physical preparations were done the previous night. Words of comfort from my daily devotional settled my heart even though I was nervous and scared about the day's surgical procedure. My family and I prayed before we left for the hospital. As we were driving, I texted two of my prayer partners and told them about the surgery and solicited their prayers. One of them called in search of a more detailed explanation. I explained the situation and she responded much like everyone else; shocked, uncertain, and in disbelief. We ended the call with a word of prayer and a promise to keep her informed.

I then thought of my brother and the many attempts to reach him. I had yet to update him on the happenings. I'd make yet another attempt to call him, this time he answered. When I told him what was going on, he became upset, and his response had a domino effect because I also became upset and began to cry. I tried to console and calm him down while trying to keep calm myself. After all, I was about to have my body opened up in surgery.

My husband, the protector, knew this was not the way that I should be just before surgery. He retrieved the phone and quickly finished the conversation with my brother. However, I had already shifted the concern for myself to my brother. I continued to give myself pep talks to get through the mind battle, "I'll be alright. I can do this," I told myself. We arrived at the hospital, I gathered my things, then we held hands and prayed again. With each step I took towards the building, I reminded myself that God was still in charge.

Faith under fire

I went directly to the surgical area for check in. I participated in the familiar routine that I had been acclimated into over the past few weeks. Checked in, verified, and the dreaded wait. The door opened and the nurse called my name and we moved at a slow pace to meet her. As we got to the door, we were greeted by the nurse and led to the room. Patient information was verified as she briefed us about the order of the day. The proper protocols were performed, vitals, blood draws, probing questions, the usual.

The nurse returned to the room to continue her assessment. She spoke with my husband and son as she continued her work. I understand that she made conversation to shift our focus from the worry associated with the surgery. When she pressed the cold stethoscope to my chest and began to listen to the rapid lub dub of my heart's rhythm, she asked, "Are you ok?" "Yes," I replied. She said, "You appear relaxed, but your heartbeat says otherwise." I smiled and said, "I am just nervous and thinking about my brother." Her many attempts to calm and reassure me led her to share her story.

Thirty-one years ago, she received a diagnosis of breast cancer while she was pregnant. Her story ended with a successful surgery and the birth of a healthy baby girl. Until this day she remains cancer free. "After today", she said, "the cancer will be left in a jar on the shelf." I appreciated her story as it gave me the encouragement I needed in that moment. I could see hope return to the faces of the men in my life. I took the time to give God a shout of praise for sending exactly what we needed.

The technician came to the room to transport me to radiology. Dr. Hunter ordered a check of my sentinel nodes to identify the exact location of the cancer. As I was wheeled through the halls, I noticed the dim lights in the hallway. We made it to the exam room where I was placed in front of an X-Ray machine that had a bed-like structure. It was unfamiliar to me.

The room felt relentlessly cold as I climbed up on the hard examination table. The iciness of the table caused me to visibly shake, so the technician offered me a warm blanket. Then the exam started. The table moved up and down as the machine took images of the affected area. After the imaging was completed, I was transferred to the attending radiologist. I received an injection of the radioactive dye which highlighted the cancerous areas. My nerves got the best of me; I felt alone, anxious, and undeniably afraid.

During this time of vulnerability, I had time to study the mannerisms of everyone I came in contact with. So far, everyone seemed to be patient, caring, and attentive. Well, that is until we got to the Radiologist. He definitely would have benefitted from taking another course in bedside manner. He never introduced himself, he did not carry on a conversation, nor did he make me feel comfortable. He just did the job and left the room. I was slightly disappointed because my experience had been full of positive interactions before meeting him.

I was transported to another area of the radiology department. There, I was greeted by two different radiologists for another series of tests. I sat in observance as they compared the various images. They explained they would need to place markers around the tumors in my breast to assist the doctor with visual parameters during the surgery. The area was numbed, and the markers were placed. After that procedure, I went back to my room to wait for the next thing on the agenda.

The nurse notified my family when I returned to the room. My husband and son walked into the room, and we watched television while we waited. Then the phone rang. It was my oldest son, Cedric, facetiming to check on me. Jacques gave him the rundown. Cedric's entire countenance dropped. He apologized profusely, as my oldest son he's always felt the need to protect me. Cedric was on a family trip, and he would have changed his plans to be there for me if I'd allowed him to. However, I told him to enjoy his family and try not to worry too much about me. His face told me he wasn't buying my "Superwoman speech." He really wanted to be with me, but cancer had interrupted our lives enough and we were determined to enjoy life. Every day was a miraculous gift.

Dr. Hunter entered the room in between surgical cases. She performed the initial assessment then notified me of my upcoming place in line. She asked if we had any questions, but we had none. My family continued to answer calls and texts while we waited. I had to be extra careful with movements because of the metal markers in place. I tried my best to relax, so I closed my eyes in an effort to feel at peace. The anesthesiologist later entered the room to give me the measured dosage, then the nurse came right behind him with medication that would ease the effects of the anesthesia. Finally, it was surgery time!

When the operating nurses entered the room, I embraced my husband and son as the nurses prepared to transport me to the operating room. The nurse placed a surgical cap on my head and off we went. As I motioned passed the nurse's desk, I was able to catch a glimpse of the brightest sunlight peering through the window.

As I reflected on the light, I was reminded of hope that I carried in my heart. We turned the corner and entered the sterile, white, and cold medical room. It was full of equipment, tools, resources, and the surgical team. There was a total of five medical professionals assigned to my surgery. Five is the number of grace. I knew grace and mercy were with me at that moment!

Everything seemed to happen so fast. The last thing I remembered was being transferred to the operating table and then I remember hearing the voices around me. The next thing I knew, I was awakened by someone calling my name. I opened my eyes and just like that, I was in recovery. The nurse asked if I was having any pain. I could not speak right then, but I motioned my head to signal no. I was unsure of how long the surgery actually lasted or how long I had been in the recovery room, all I knew was that I was alive and hopefully left all the cancer in a jar on the shelf. I was taken to the post-op room to get settled in.

Once settled, the nurse allowed my family in. My husband and son entered the room. I was still a little drowsy from the anesthesia, but I remember my husband made a comment on how well the surgery went. I met all the criteria for discharge. While waiting for the counsel in the discharge instructions, I had a visitor, my pastor's wife. I was so happy to see her and hear her voice.

As the nurse was inspecting my incision, I could see the First Lady looking over her shoulder. I smiled, knowing she was my prayer warrior and yet another angel God assigned to me. After the nurse presented the discharge instructions, my husband helped me get dressed and we were out of there! I thanked the nurse again for sharing her story and for the great care she provided. She transported me to my vehicle from the wheelchair, helped me inside, and insistently said, "now go tell your story," I smiled and nodded my head in appreciation as she closed the door.

Chapter 4

Participate in the Plan

My surgery was over, but the waiting felt like an eternity. Based on the results from my biopsy and images, the doctors knew the cancer was DCIS and the next round of treatment would include radiation. Further examination of the mass would determine my treatment.

When I returned home from surgery, I rested as much as possible. I was grateful that my pain was minimal… I was careful not to pull or tug at my bandages as I shifted from side to side in bed.

Later that evening, my nephew arrived from college. He was the last close family member that was unaware of my diagnosis. I was watching television in my room when he crept into the room and hugged me. However, our embrace was different this time. As he leaned in towards me, I mentioned to him that I had just had surgery. He stood up and looked intensely at me and asked, "Are you OK?" I shared with him the diagnosis of breast cancer and explained the type of procedure that was done. I explained to him that

I did not want him to worry about me while he focused on his studies. I assured him I'd be alright.

I've experienced certain situations in which people have shared their cancer survival stories that attracted the wrong attention. Those who hear the stories often pity, are overly compassionate, or feel sorry for the individual. I did not want anyone's pity. I just needed their prayers. I knew if I remained positive, I'd get through *this* victoriously.

I struggled with overthinking. It was easy for me to slip into negative thinking, but I didn't want my attitude to dictate my actions. Thankfully, I am humble enough to take a personal inventory and identify my area of weakness. I knew I could not battle this on my own, so there were select people that I trusted to war with me. A team of divine prayer warriors. This battle had to be fought strategically! Not only did I request specific prayer, but I also wrote and read scriptures to keep me strengthened. I posted positive affirmations everywhere. They were in my bedroom, bathroom, the living room, and every other place I accessed.

I was required to suit up spiritually, physically, and mentally daily. And I struggled day by day! However, I am thankful for the prayers of my family and friends. Their prayers helped carry me through rough times.

I continued on the road to recovery after surgery to prepare my body for the next phase. I took time and researched breast cancer because radiation was a part of the treatment. One day while I was researching, my phone rang. The number on the caller ID read "unknown." The clerk at Dr. Hunter's office alerted me that if I received a call from an unknown number, then most likely it was the clinic or hospital. I quickly answered the call. It was Dr. Hunter. She verified her identity then asked about my well-being. I explained to her how I felt, then she proceeded with the matter at hand. She confirmed that my follow up appointment was only a few days away; however, she called to provide the results of my testing.

I tried to jot down everything she said. The results confirmed the DCIS, but it also revealed something else. There was a small area the size of a pen head that showed Invasive Cancer. When those words fell from her lips, I felt my heart palpitate and my respirations were labored. Dr. Hunter stated that my Sentinel lymph nodes and margins were all clear and the cancer had not spread. However, she was unsure of Dr. Garza's treatment plan. I had a million and one questions, and the reality of fighting cancer was frightening but my faith increased. I expected God to heal me.

I called Charles into the bedroom and told him what the doctor said. I felt his loving concern as he sat on the bed next to me. He held my hands tightly and said, "We got this!" After he left the room, I searched the internet for information on Invasive Cancer. The more information I read the more anxious I became. I put the searching on pause because I felt the need to pray. Journaling and praying were my therapy.

When I felt like my mind was overloaded, I went to my quiet place to meditate, pray, and journal. My journal is filled with prayers, praise reports, and prophetic words. As I looked back over the written words, I praised God for His faithfulness. Every promise He made to me during the midnight of my life has manifested.

I didn't return to work until weeks after the surgery. The recovery time was only set for a few days; however, I took a little extra time to relax and further process my situation. My family took great care of me during my recovery. Finally, the time had come for my follow up with Dr. Hunter. Everything was going well, and the surgical site healed beautifully. My visit with Dr. Hunter was pleasant as she and her staff showed genuine care and concern for me. Later that month, I was scheduled to visit Dr. Garza for her to also assess my recovery.

Although my husband was a pillar of strength, there were times when he needed to be strengthened as well. He contacted our pastor and a friend to share how he felt. He was referred to a few couples who had gone through their battle with cancer as well. The very thought of contacting people that we didn't know was nerve wrecking; but we needed a village of people to help us. Thankfully, they were open to conversation. There was an instant connection with the first couple we called… Our stories were very similar. The wife was in her third year of remission and radiation therapy wasn't necessary. This talk helped me more than I could have imagined. She understood my fear and anxiety perfectly. I felt refreshed after the call, especially when she prayed with me.

A few days later, I contacted the second person, but I was still nervous. This beautiful soul was friends with our Pastor and First Lady, so we started our conversation with that common bond. I shared my story with her and where I was in the process. She began to tell me her story. As she shared, I wrote down one specific thing she stated. She told me how she had received a promotion on her job and was on a business trip when she received a call to return home. She shared how she stepped away from her dream job to fight cancer and live. I felt an instant connection with her because her story was similar to mine.

I also received a promotion in February 2017. It was my dream job, but shortly after I received a diagnosis of breast cancer. We continued to talk for a few more minutes. Our conversation flowed like we have known each other for years. She was a three-year breast cancer survivor.

Those calls took me out of my comfort zone, but I needed these divine connections. Even to this day, I remain in contact with my shero, her name is Shaun Bailey. We have developed a bond and I am thankful that God connected our paths. We have an inside joke and tell people we are "breast friends." I heard many say I was so secretive during my breast cancer journey, but I say it was strategy not secrecy.

There are times in life when everyone should not be privy to certain information or even have access to us or our situation. This is a time when we need to create an atmosphere that is conducive for our needs. Fortunately, not everyone makes the cut! As I prayed and sought God, He placed the right people in my life. I believed God answered both of our prayers and blessed us with an eternal friendship.

Time progressed, and we were approaching Memorial Day weekend. Many of our close friends celebrated the graduations of their children and/or grandchildren. I scrolled through Facebook in admiration of their joyfulness. We celebrated with our own victories at our home. Charles put together a backyard bar-b-que and we spent quality time as a family. I recalled the times that I wanted to give up but images of us making beautiful memories together flooded my mind. I did not want those memory making moments to end, so each day I fought a little harder.

The time had come for my return to work. When I arrived for the morning report, the room was filled with laughter and smiling faces. For a Monday morning everyone was quite lively. We completed our morning report and a few of my peers asked how I was doing. We chatted for a few moments, and I happily shared my testimony of good health. I spent most of my time catching up on emails and attending meetings. It felt good to be back to work, but something was slightly off. Something about this once normal routine felt extremely different!

The next morning, I went to the Cancer Center for an appointment with Dr. Garza. I felt scared and nervous… Although, this was the same routine I had rehearsed many times before. Check in, wait, call back, exam room, in that order. Dr. Garza entered the room shortly after I was directed back. She greeted my husband and I, then went right into the review of my results. When she began speaking, I was attentive and intentional as I did not want to miss or misinterpret any of the information that she'd share. Dr. Garza expressed her dissatisfaction with the margins after careful review. Therefore, she recommended another surgery to remove more breast tissue to ensure that all cancer was gone.

Anger and fear consumed me as I listened to the words spill from her lips. To add insult to injury, she also shared the results of the genetic screening that showed high-risk for ovarian cancer, too. Not only did I need another surgery to remove MORE breast tissue, but also, a recommended surgery to remove my ovaries too! Wait! What? God, got to be kidding! I needed to scream and a loud inner-voice told me to run out of that room. From that point, doubt crept in, and I became uncertain regarding every decision I had made. I felt myself losing it. Before I knew it, I belted out, "I want a double mastectomy!"

Dr. Garza appeared shocked at my declaration, but I did not want to keep subjecting myself to the pain and anguish of surgery and recovery. She agreed with my decision and informed me of next steps in the new plan. As Dr. Garza continued with the visit and began the examination, something amazing happened! The doctor placed her hand on my right shoulder and asked me to take a deep breath as she listened to my heart and breathing pattern. This normal protocol seemed as if it had been hijacked by God. The doctor took longer than usual to listen. She remained in that same position at least double the normal time. During that exchange, I felt my nerves calm and my fear subsided. God's peace that comforted me. I never asked Dr. Garza to confirm, but I believed God directed her to prayer.

After the exam, she informed me that the Cancer Tumor Board was scheduled to meet that evening and my case would be discussed. Dr. Hunter was a member of the board, and she would include my decision for a double mastectomy in the conversation. As we closed the visit, Dr. Garza said, "It will be alright." I didn't know to what degree I believed *that* anymore. As we drove home, Charles and I were silent. I was still trying to process what happened.

When we arrived home, I retreated to my quiet place. I had a lot to think about. That news crushed my spirit. I was thankful for Dr. Garza. Even though I didn't get the report that I'd hoped for, I felt she truly cared and was genuinely concerned for my health. With new risk factors involved, I was faced with the challenge to search for a gynecologist.

Another appointment with Dr. Hunter was scheduled within the next few days. At the appointment she shared the discussion that the board had concerning my case. Since a double mastectomy procedure was on the table, she provided literature for me to read. We also discussed setting a date for a dual surgery. I wanted to get everything done at once to get it over with. I asked if it were possible to perform the double mastectomy and hysterectomy at the same time. The answer was yes. The problem was, I had not yet chosen a provider. She gave her recommendation, and we went from there. We agreed that I would first make an appointment with the GYN clinic she suggested, then they could move forward and coordinate a surgery date. Reconstruction surgery came up again in the discussion. But yet again, this was not something that I was ready to talk about.

Later that day, I scheduled the GYN appointment. During the screening I realized that it had been some time since my last Pap. May as well throw that appointment in there too while I'm at it. The pap smear appointment was successful. I was able to catch up with the business of old colleagues. I also had an opportunity to share my story with the nurse. Her daughter was going through cancer treatments, and this was my opportunity to encourage her as she encouraged me.

By now, it was mid-June 2017. I thought radiation treatments would have started and almost completed according to the original plan. One appointment after another had become my new normal. The next schedule on the agenda was the GYN.

I arrived at the clinic with copies of my medical records in hand. I wanted to be prepared to keep things moving forward. Dr. Meza was the new face to the sea of doctors that were on my plan of care. During the visit, he reviewed my medical history and asked about recent gynecological procedures. He continued to probe for more answers about my health history before he mentioned a plan to move forward with surgery. He informed me he would get with Dr. Hunter to coordinate a surgery date. The plan consisted of Dr. Hunter first performing the double mastectomy, then Dr. Meza to come in right after to perform the hysterectomy. The plan sounded good, I just don't know how prepared I was or would be when that time came.

Well into the summer months, many people took vacations and were out of the office, so it wasn't as busy. A week or so passed before I received a call from Dr. Hunter's office to schedule an appointment for the confirmation of my surgery date. After all, I looked forward to those visits with her. By now, I had enough time to think about that reconstructive surgery that she kept bringing up. It was more of a consideration than an afterthought at this point. At first, I didn't consider the change a double mastectomy brought with it. Later that evening, I shared my consideration of reconstructive surgery with my husband for feedback. He just simply stated that he would pray that I made the best decision for me. This led me to research information on breast reconstructive surgery to help me to make a well-informed decision.

In my research many questions arose, since there was no one there that could answer my inquiries immediately, I made a list to ask Dr. Hunter at my next visit. The appointment with Dr. Hunter was set to finalize the surgery. As we talked, I mentioned that I was considering reconstructive surgery. She provided the name of a physician out of Edmond, OK. He visited Lawton, OK twice a month to see patients. I agreed to set up an appointment with the provider. Because of this newly introduced consideration, the surgery date that was set to be finalized had to be postponed.

A week later, I was scheduled to see the Plastic Surgeon to discuss breast reconstructive surgery. I was able to see the doctor at the Lawton location, which was located in Dr. Hunter's office as well. My husband and I arrived at the appointment. Both of us were nervous and unsure about what to expect. The nurse escorted us to the exam room to see the doctor. Then Dr. Panchal entered the room. He was dressed in a navy-blue suit and carried himself in a very professional manner. He was a sharp doctor and I perceived that he was passionate about what he did. He introduced himself to Charles and I and asked what my line of work was. I told him I was a Registered Nurse and I worked at the Oklahoma City VA. He began to call off names of doctors he knew that worked at the hospital. I appreciated his friendly demeanor, it helped me relax for the appointment.

Dr. Panchal provided a plethora of informational resources on breast reconstruction. I shared with him my plans of having all surgeries performed one after the other on the same day. With all the surgeries, double mastectomy, reconstructive surgery, and hysterectomy; the total surgery time would be approximately six hours. Charles and I looked at each other disapprovingly after we heard that. Our visit concluded with all this information; I had a lot to think about.

After long deliberation and educating myself through the process, I decided to go through with the reconstructive surgery. My only concern was the lengthy surgical time… SIX hours! I was not sure if my body could handle six hours of cutting, poking, and prodding. I called Dr. Panchal's office to confirm my decision. Another appointment was scheduled to begin the process.

At that appointment, I shared my concerns with Dr. Panchal. I mentioned the lengthy process of the combined surgeries. He advised me to focus on the breasts first, the main thing was to remove all cancer and restore the breasts. The other surgery is a risk, but no cancer was found in that area. That surgery could be revisited at a later date. His advice was very reasonable, and it made sense to accept such a practical solution.

The decision was made to postpone the hysterectomy. With that off the schedule, the surgery time was reduced to four hours instead of six. The procedures went as follows: Dr. Hunter would start the surgery and once she was completed, Dr. Panchal would come in to insert the tissue expanders. "Tissue expanders are temporary, expandable, balloon-like devices used after mastectomy to stretch skin and chest wall muscles so that the breast implants can be adequately accommodated." (Article Causes and Management of Tissue Expander Pain. Pam Stephan, May 14, 2020.). This surgery would require an overnight stay, but if there were no complications, I could be released as early as the next day.

While I was waiting to hear from Dr. Hunter's office, I received a call from Dr. Meza's with a date for surgery. I was confused by the call, but I quickly realized Dr. Meza's office was not aware of the change in plans. I informed the nurse of my updated decision and told her I would follow up with Dr. Meza after my other surgery. That surgery date was finalized for August 7, 2017.

Mid-July arrived and we finally had a solidified plan and surgery date. July is the month our family celebrated the

McKire Family reunion in Florida. This year was a special year for our family, as my Uncle Howard and Aunt Vera would celebrate their 60th Wedding Anniversary in August of 2017. As one of the vice chairs for our family reunion, I suggested we highlight their milestone for our banquet night. The event was planned in June just in case I was not able to travel to Florida for the reunion. With my surgery date scheduled for August, I had time to be with my family during the celebration. My husband agreed and we quickly made arrangements with our jobs and flights to travel home during that time.

We arrived in Florida and the team met to finalize plans for our Saturday event. After the meeting, we grabbed a quick lunch. My brother joined Charles and I, and he didn't waste any time asking the plethora of questions that plagued his mind about my health. I answered his questions to the best of my ability and ended the conversation as I usually did, "But… I'll be fine." Being back home with family for a few days allowed me to take my mind off of my illness and enjoy the time I spent with my family.

Our family reunion started that Friday night with a fish fry. It was nice to see my family members come together, especially ones that I hadn't seen in a while. My Uncle graced me with the task of opening up the reunion with prayer. It was my honor to do so.

The beauty of living in a small town is that people from the community often stopped in to help us celebrate family. A great time was had by all. Food, family, and fellowship was the perceived mantra. I really needed this time with my family to relax and have fun. The next morning some of my family went to Cracker Barrel for breakfast. We had an amazing time together. As I looked at each of them, I intentionally cherished our time together. I was very cognizant of the fact that I didn't know when we would spend time together again.

Banquet time! Charles and I arrived early to make sure the decorations and other items were good to go. We held the event at the Lake City Country Club, where my brother Johnny works. We walked in and I was overjoyed with how beautiful the room looked. The decorator made sure to capture every little detail that was described to her. I knew my Uncle and Aunt were going to love what we had planned for them. The cakes and cupcakes were delivered and set up. Beautiful work was done by all. Then my family members started to arrive. As they entered the building, we captured photos of everyone mingling as they raved over about décor.

When Uncle Howard and Aunt Vera arrived, I met them at the door, gave them their gift, and captured some pictures before they went inside. While I was outside stalling, my husband was busy inside gathering the family so they would be ready.

As my aunt and uncle walked into the room, they were met with a standing ovation, loud cheers, and applause. The look on their faces at that moment was priceless. Cameras flashed as they walked through embracing others and sharing love. It was a beautifully unforgettable moment. In spite of everything I had faced from April until then, this moment was everything I needed. Love, laughter, and family are truly the best forms of medicine.

We ate, laughed, danced, and sang the whole night long. One part of the program allowed everyone to share special words with Uncle Howard and Aunt Vera. When my time came to share, I couldn't decide what I wanted to say. The most pressing thing on my mind was whether or not I should share my condition with the family. As I started to share how much my uncle and aunt meant to me and their support to me and my brothers during the passing of our mother, I could no longer hold the secret that I had kept. So, I confessed my struggle.

As I shared, I looked around the room and some had looks of shock and others wiped away tears. My Uncle Joseph, my mother's oldest sibling, was recording the event. I turned around to him walking towards me with his hand out to pray. Everything stopped and went silent. The family joined hands and they stood in the gap for me. My cousin Ricky, who is a Pastor, stood with my Uncle Joseph as he prayed over me. When my uncle finished the prayer, he directed us all to recite Psalms 23 in its entirety. I can only imagine what my Uncles were thinking as only 6 years ago, they heard the same diagnosis for their sister, and my mother, who is no longer with us. My cousin, who was a breast cancer survivor, embraced me and told me if I had any questions to contact her.

To liven up the atmosphere after that super emotional moment, my husband grabbed the microphone and told a joke. I can't even remember what he said… but it was enough to make us laugh! We continued on with our event and had a great time. Throughout the evening, family members came up to me and gave hugs and words of encouragement. After sharing with the rest of my family, I felt much less burdened.

The next morning, we attended church together as a family. The service was great. The last day of our family reunion included a trip to the beach. We barbecued, swam, and played games. This year was very special to me. Usually, one of my siblings is unable to make it. But this time the whole gang showed up. I enjoyed every minute of our time together. I danced, rode on the boat, and cheered for everyone who tried their luck at horseshoes. Making memories and basking in the love of my family was the highlight of that weekend. We ended our reunion like always with our family doing a count off of everyone in attendance and closing in prayer.

Charles and I headed to the airport for an early flight back to Oklahoma. I looked through my IPAD at the many pictures we took during the reunion. I felt so blessed to have my family. I knew the days ahead would be busy, but I wanted this moment to last a little while longer. We safely arrived back home in Lawton, OK and jumped back into our regularly scheduled program. With surgeries and other appointments quickly approaching, I tried to put in as much work as possible. I had so many things to close out before my surgery. My recovery time would be approximately three weeks. I knew I needed to make a trip to one of the clinics I supervised to share the news with the staff. Prior to my promotion, I was the Nurse Manager for this clinic for three years.

As a work family, we were very close knit. I scheduled a visit to the clinic on Thursday. After the morning huddle, I shared with the staff, I had breast cancer and I was going to have surgery the following week. Some of the staff began to cry while others stood in line to hug me. They all shared words of encouragement and before ending our huddle, they said a prayer for me. I stayed at the clinic all day to spend time with them and help answer any questions they had.

The weekend before my surgery was my birthday, July 29, 2017. The morning of my birthday, I woke up and praised God for allowing me to see another birthday. A few months earlier, I had questioned if I would live to see my 48th birthday. Charles planned a nice weekend getaway to

Dallas, TX. Usually, I was the one who planned our trips, but this year I had no idea of what to expect.

To my surprise, it turned out to be pretty great. We saw a play, shopped, and ate at new restaurants. Even though the festivities were centered around my birthday, I knew this was a much-needed break for Charles as well. He had been so attentive, so giving, and so patient. His support assured me that I was not in this alone. I was not the only one that was going through this, but he walked with me every step of the way.

Chapter 5

Embrace Hope

The days that led up to the surgery were very busy. I wanted to make sure everything was in order… *just in case.* I realized that updated beneficiary information to the life insurance policies had not adjusted for quite some time. I figured this was as good a time as any to get that done. It's not that I had any doubts that I would come out of surgery and be just fine, but it's smart to keep things up to date as a precaution. That task opened me up to questions that I really didn't want swimming in my head. I had to think of how to disburse an equal distribution of funds to my family if something were to happen to me. The very thought that something could possibly happen to me sooner than expected brought feelings of fear and angst.

Next on the docket was to get my hair done. I knew my movement would be limited and grooming tasks would be quite difficult. So, I chose a low maintenance braid style to get me through this moderately stationary period. My beautician coordinated with another stylist and braided my hair to perfection. She was such an inspiration to me during my journey. Her first response was to pray when I revealed my illness. I am thankful that I had people strategically placed in my life who prayed for me! This is priceless.

There were still a few things I had to solidify before I went on medical leave. During my rounds to the different clinics, I went to my friend Kathleen's office. We sat and had a lively conversation about work and family and ended it with prayer. As Kathleen prayed, tears fell from my eyes like fresh rain in early Spring. Every word was heartfelt and resonated in the parts of my soul that needed it the most. She has been a true warrior that keeps me connected. She seemed to know just when to send up a powerful prayer, an encouraging text, or a perfect scripture to fit my situation… These irreplaceable acts of love got me through many days.

My workday ended and I gathered my belongings to leave for an undetermined amount of time. As I walked to my car, I looked back at the hospital and wondered, "Will I ever return?"

As I sat in the beauty shop waiting my turn, my daughter in law called me on Facetime with my granddaughter, Alicia. I answered quickly, eager to see that cute little face of hers. As soon as she saw my face, she yelled "Hello Nana!" I replied "Hello Alicia. Happy Birthday!" She was so excited to tell me about all the great gifts she received, but I was not long on the phone before the stylist gave the ready signal to start on my hair. I told her that I loved her, and I would call her back later. The busy day finally ended. I returned home to have dinner and a relaxing night with my husband.

On Saturday morning I slept in. Friday was so busy I was not eager to move around early. Later that afternoon, I went shopping to get all the essentials post-surgery. My sons returned to school to resume their studies. They came back the day before the surgery, they wouldn't have been any other place!

We went to Church on Sunday and really enjoyed the service. During prayer time, our Pastor and First Lady prayed with me and Charles. I cried most of the time. The prayer, praise, worship, and the sermon charged the atmosphere. I felt such peace as I sat in the service. It was as if God was sitting right next to me, and His presence reassured me that I was never alone… Even in this moment.

Later that evening, I tried to relax and watch some of my favorite television shows. I couldn't help but to think about the life changing event that was about to take place. As I prepared for my shower, I slowly turned to face the mirror. I looked down at my breast… sadly, I thought… I am losing part of me. I even took pictures of them to remind me of what I looked like before this dreaded fate. I cried as I struggled to understand and said, "God, why is this happening to me?" Of course, I am not defined by my body parts, but when parts that were once there are no longer there because of a cruel uncontrollable disease; confusion, anger, grief, and hopelessness are inevitable. I had a "Lord please take this cup away from me moment. But, nevertheless, let your will be done." I knew I would eventually be A BETTER me. So, I said my goodbyes… And I kept hope alive!

August 7, 2017, surgery day finally arrived. This day started just as other days, with prayer and devotion. We then prepared to take the long trip to the hospital. The boys were in one car and Charles, and I were in another. They were permitted to miss that day from practice at camp to be there with me for surgery. However, when I got the "ok" clearance after surgery, they would head back. We arrived at the hospital, got registered, went through all the preliminaries, and then the wait began. While waiting, we busied ourselves to pass the time and ease our nerves. My husband and I turned our attention to the morning news, while our boys entertained themselves scrolling through social media.

The long wait did not help with my anxiety. The longer we sat the more nervous I became. My legs told the story as they restlessly bounced up and down. Suddenly, my name was called. I walked towards the door with my husband and boys in tow. Initially, my husband was the only one allowed to accompany me to the back. When I got to the room, I suited up in the required gear to perform the assessment and surgery prep.

Dr. Hunter entered the room wearing a radiant and comforting smile. She explained the procedure for the day and gave an opportunity for questions. There were a few cases scheduled ahead of mine that afforded a little more downtime.

As we waited, Dr. Panchal visited my room. I was so accustomed to seeing him in suits, but this time he wore surgical scrubs. He completed his assessment and gave me a compliment. Before he left the room, he charged Charles with the task of taking good care of me. I continued to watch television and answer texts from family members, while I waited. Since there was still some time before surgery, the nurse allowed my boys to come back to the room.

Now, it was time for surgery. The nurses came with the wheelchair to escort me. I kissed and hugged Charles and the boys and told them I loved them before I made my way out of the room. I could sense the nervousness within them because I felt the same thing. When I reached the operating room and was transferred to the operating table, I was overwhelmed by the most intense feeling of fear. I was scheduled for a four-hour surgery and had no idea what the outcome would be. I tried hard to erase the possibilities of death from my mind. I could hear the chatter of the doctors and nurses around me. I focused on the Anesthesiologist as he explained to me the effects of the medication that he administered. I nodded in agreement and the next thing I knew I was awakened to someone encouraging me to eat. I opened my eyes to Charles, my boys, and our friends, the Aldridge's at my bedside.

I did not remember anything between the anesthesia and the moment I opened my eyes. I had very little pain, but I was extremely drowsy. I was in and out of consciousness. I was awake one minute and asleep the next. When I did fall asleep, I was awakened to the sound of Joanne, "You need to eat". She fed me little bites to eat the dish on my bed tray. In the midst of all of that, it was getting late, and my boys had to get back on the road to school. They said their goodbyes and headed out.

Anthony and Joanne are family friends. We met them at church in Lawton, OK in 2003. Joanne and I quickly developed a relationship. One day Joanne and I attended a Women's Fellowship. We participated in an ice breaker exercise in which we had to tell one thing we liked about the person next to us. Joanne shared that I was nice, quiet, and that she admired me because of my consistent prayer life. We never know who is watching us, so we should always be the best version of ourselves. Joanne's words blessed my heart and from that moment our friendship blossomed beautifully.

My husband was deployed to Iraq at that time. While he was away, I was an acting single parent in a new town with two school aged children in school. My family and support system were hundreds of miles away in Florida. Having to learn a new city, a new job, join a new church, and find a new support system seemed impossible and overwhelming simultaneously. My connection to Joanne was vital during this time of my life. I appreciated her then and I appreciate her even more now.

By now, I was stuffed from Joanne force feeding me. I could not eat one more bite. All I wanted at this point was to get more sleep. Joanne and Anthony prepared to leave so I could do just that, sleep. After they left, Charles and I talked a little before we both were too tired to keep our eyes opened. Charles tried hard to find a comfortable position to sleep with the one-star hospital guest accommodations. But somehow, he managed to get a little rest.

The next morning, I received a visit from Dr. Hunter. She completed her assessment and informed me that I'd be discharged later that day. She encouraged me to take it easy and to call the clinic if I had any questions or concerns. I was ready to go home. My first time out of bed was a little difficult. The nurse helped me prepare to leave. I was a little dizzy from the medication, but thankful it was nothing more. There were also four tubes inserted in my chest to allow fluid drainage from the surgery area. The tubes needed to be drained periodically. To ensure that it was done properly, Dr. Hunter ordered a home health nurse for assistance with the tubes and dressing changes. Being a registered nurse, I was skilled in performing these tasks, but of course, not on myself.

While having to do things in slow motion, I had time to carefully perform a self-examination. I studied the area of my chest where my original breasts once were and discovered two padded bandages. I wondered what it would look like when the bandages came off. As surprising as it might sound, I was in no pain. Of course, I had strong medication to help manage that, but it surprised me. I needed Charles' help to do simple things like getting in and out of the bed. I also had to learn to do things on my own with limited range of motion. That was quite the challenge, but I was up for it.

After breakfast, I was ready to go. The nurse disconnected the IV and powered down the monitors. Charles assisted me in getting dressed while the nurse completed the discharge paperwork. Our boys called to check in just before we left. Seeing their faces through Facetime gave my heart such joy. They were thrilled to know that I was released from the hospital. I was excited to go but was also terrified. Was I leaving too soon? What if something bad happens while I'm at home? Questions like these bombarded my mind as I rolled through the hallways of the hospital to exit. Nonetheless, I pressed on.

We made it safely to our home, and Charles ensured that I was comfortable and properly cared for. He helped to get me dressed and undressed, he propped my pillow for my comfort, and he administered my pain medication. He did everything I needed to ensure that I was totally comfortable. He wanted me to rest… And I did. I slept for a while. Then Charles awakened me to do a wellness check. I decided I wanted to get out of bed and go into the living room to watch television.

While sitting quietly, I received a phone call from my son Cedric and a visit from our friends Anthony and Joanne. Cedric was unable to be present during the surgery because he could not take time off from the military and school. I could hear concern in his voice as he wanted to make sure that I was okay.

Anthony and Joann brought us dinner for the evening. After we greeted them, we sat down and ate together. I felt the urge to use the restroom and Charles assisted me. Suddenly, I felt as if something had popped inside my chest. I grabbed the left side of my chest as delicately as I could to ease the pain. Then I told Charles, "Something doesn't feel right." We checked the bandages, the drains, and the tubing. Everything appeared to be as it should. We sat down to eat. While we were conversing with our friend, I felt a swelling sensation in my chest. I thought it was all in my head and I didn't want to overact. So, I carried on as if nothing was wrong. Then, I felt a rising in my chest. I yelled out, "My chest is swelling, something is not right." Charles rushed to get me to the hospital.

He was extremely frantic, and he considered taking me to the fire station in hopes of quicker care. I assured him that it was fine for him to get me to the emergency room.

When we arrived, Charles parked by the front door and ran inside. I sat quietly in the truck as I fought my fears and attempted to restrain my tears. Charles came back to the truck with assistance, and I was immediately treated. The nurse took my vitals and asked routine questions. One of the nurses was concerned about Charles and asked about his well-being. I knew my husband wasn't okay because I wasn't okay. I was afraid, actually more terrified! I thought I was going to die. I wasn't ready and my faith wouldn't let me believe this was my expected end. I had to KEEP H.O.P.E. alive!

Charles was escorted to my room. I could tell he had been crying… I wanted to hold him and reassure him that I was fine, but at that point uncertainty attempted to consume me. The doctor came into the room, asking more questions and assessing my chest area. The doctor gave the nurses orders to draw blood, take rectal temperature and contact the General Surgery Provider on call. Of all the evenings to have student nurses in the emergency room, I figured tonight was not a good time. My anxiety skyrocketed!

Charles called our pastor, and he came to pray. He declared the Word of God and LIFE over me. I needed GOD's peace desperately at that moment. It was difficult to remain calm, the student nurses struggled to perform simple tasks. Taking my temperature was a tedious task for them, if I wasn't in so much pain, I would have done it myself! Eventually the lead nurse came to my room and completed my assessment. I threw my hands up in my head in pure gratitude!

By now the pain in my chest had gotten more intense and I was afraid to move. The doctor advised that I be admitted and treated for infection. I was not convinced that I had an infection, but I was too exhausted to object; I simply agreed to stay. When I arrived on my assigned floor, I needed to use the restroom. As soon as I stood to wash my hands, I felt lightheaded and faint. I knew I was about to fall. The nurse saved me before I hit the floor. She assisted me into the wheelchair and ordered that I should call for assistance before getting out of the bed. The nurse ensured I was back in bed safely and ordered fall precautions.

Charles returned to the house to pack a bag for our stay. He seemed a little calmer, but he couldn't hide the pain of not being able to heal me. I wanted so badly to fall asleep, but I was afraid I would not wake up. To add insult to injury, there was a noisy patient on our floor. The patient yelled all night long. The nurse closed my door to minimize the noise, but I could still hear them. Hospitals have the perceived expectation of quiet, but this was not what I expected at all. Being behind closed doors made me even more fearful than I had been before. I hoped that Charles would hurry back!

Charles finally made it back and pulled the recliner next to my bed to help me relax. After a few hours, the nurse came in to do another assessment. She pressed the affected area on my chest, and I immediately grabbed her hand. I thought that she was handling me a little too rough. She apologized but I didn't believe it was genuine, but I restrained myself from being rude. She administered pain medication and I started to relax. As I laid in the bed, I watched the clock as the night transitioned into day.

I looked out of the window and the moon light shined so brightly that it held my attention for the entire night. The light was my guide. I told myself, if I make it to 5:00 AM, I will be alright. I reflected back to that moment in my journey when I cried out to God on the floor of the hotel bathroom. In that I was directed to the scripture 2 Corinthians 12:9 that reads, *"My grace is sufficient for you, for My strength is made perfect in weakness."* I needed so much to believe this. As I meditated on that word, I felt such peace and reassurance I would live and not die. The outside noise was no longer a distraction, and I was able to fall asleep peacefully.

As soon as I closed my eyes, I was awakened by the heavy-handed nurse to take my vital signs. Dr. Hunter entered my room and explained that I had a hematoma on my left side; it attributed to the pain and swelling. According to Merriam-Webster, a hematoma is a mass of usually clotted blood that forms in a tissue, organ, or body space because of a broken blood vessel." The plastic surgeon needed to be informed of the happenings. Consequently, I had to return to Oklahoma City to see him. Charles and I made plans to visit Dr. Panchal's office while we waited for discharge.

The nurse arrived and to my surprise it was someone I knew from church. She handled the discharge. Although I still had swelling on the left side of my chest, I had to travel an hour and half to see Dr. Panchal. My pain was manageable, but the nurse wanted to make sure that I didn't need anything before I left. She ensured that I had enough pain medication.

Charles and I left the hospital. He stopped by our house for a pillow and blanket so I would be comfortable on the ride. I closed my eyes and laid my head back to relax. I must have fallen asleep, because when I opened my eyes, we were only a few miles from the doctor's office. The pain in my chest had intensified once again; however, I was afraid to take any medication since I hadn't eaten anything. We made it to Dr. Panchal's office and entered the building where a nurse met us and transported us to the exam room immediately. Dr. Panchal completed his exam and notified me that I would have to go into surgery... AGAIN! I was not happy at all, anger and frustration brewed within me. I desperately NEEDED this part of my story to be over...

The surgery was scheduled immediately, August 9, 2017, to be exact. We had to travel about 20 minutes to the surgery center. Once again, I was lying on the cold, hard surgery table. I couldn't help but to cry after being subjected to *this pain*, not once, not twice, but three times [so far]. I was over it!

The anesthesiologist gave me "the drowsy speech," administered the anesthesia, and then I was out. When I woke up, I was in the recovery room. The pain had subsided, and I felt much better. I was offered crackers and water and ate them with no problems. Charles later entered the room with a huge smile on his face after he looked into my eyes. I couldn't help but smile back. "How are you feeling?", he asked. "I feel so much better!? I replied. I remained in their care to be monitored a little longer. There were tubes pinned on my gown to keep them in place and the bandages were tightly secured. My mom had once prayed over a handkerchief, and she kept it close during her journey. Since it was my turn, I inherited the handkerchief and took it with me through every surgery. I told the nurse's my heirloom handkerchief was missing and although they searched for it, they didn't find it. I didn't want the loss of the handkerchief to get me down, so I refocused on recovery.

Reflecting back on the moment I lost the handkerchief; I went and bought a new pack and anointed them with oil and prayed over them… Just like my mom did when I was a little girl. I believed that my prayers and faith were powerful enough and strong enough to give me the same assurance. If it worked for my mother, I knew faith had to work for me too! At that moment, God showed me my prayers are just as anointing as my mom's prayers. My faith is a generational blessing! I know I have come this far by faith… and my mother's prayers!

We had an hour and half drive home. I felt so much better and was hungry! I told Charles I wanted a McDonald's fish sandwich. He looked at me with a smile and took me straight there. The phone was flooded with phone calls and text messages from our family requesting updates. Charles talked with one of our friends and laughed at my "McDonald's" dinner request. I had not eaten a meal for the past day and half, I was practically starving. Dr. Panchal promised after my surgery I would feel better, and I did.

As we drove home, I felt more relaxed, and I enjoyed listening to the music during the ride. We arrived home safely and prepared for bed. I tried my best to get comfortable, so I propped pillows under me and shifted positions carefully, but nothing worked.

I tried to sit in the recliner in the living room, but I could not tolerate the pulling feeling in my chest. Then, I tried the sofa and found a comfortable spot. I wanted to sleep there for the night to get some rest. Charles slept in the recliner next to me through the night.

For the next three weeks, our living room was where we slept. I had a hard time lying flat in the bed for a while. I purchased new pillows and back rests, but it was painful. I am so thankful for my husband. Seeing him sleep night after night in the recliner next to me was lovingly assuring, it's the little big things that mean EVERYTHING. I told him several times that he could sleep in the bed, but he insisted he would stay by my side. This was one of the many gestures he did that proves his unconditional love for me.

The Worst Helped Us Get Better...

Prior to my breast cancer diagnosis, Charles and I experienced some rough times in our marriage. Due to my promotion at work, I had to travel frequently, and it caused a strain on our marriage. We struggled for months to communicate effectively with each other. When our lives suddenly change and the fear of death looms at our door, the little things seem so trivial. We are not a perfect couple, but we have learned to fight for marriage and the happiness we desire. To give up on our marriage was never an option.

I wrote a prayer in my journal, and I stated, "God, please forgive Charles and I for our behavior in our marriage." I kept the prayer simple; God knew what we needed. I realized that we took our time together for granted. The day we received my diagnosis, both of us had an immediate reality check! We understood tomorrow wasn't promised to us… so we had to honor the vows we made to each other. Charles and I promised to love each other in sickness and health.

In 2016, Charles ruptured his patella tendon playing basketball. For months he underwent surgery and rehabilitation. I supported him through the entire process. Now it was his turn to care for me. For weeks after surgery, he bathed me, dressed me, emptied drains, changed bandages and so much more. We created so many positive and loving memories during one of the darkest times in our lives. I must admit, I was afraid Charles would leave me, having a wife with cancer wasn't an easy pill to swallow.

I heard so many stories from other ladies, where their spouse walked away in the middle of their cancer journey. Thankfully, this is not my story. From day one, Charles promised me he was with me forever. Today, our marriage is stronger than ever, and we are enjoying life and serving God's people together. This season helped us provide premarital and marital counseling to several couples. Again, we were reminded (in the midst of turmoil) that EVERYTHING works together for our good.

Two days after surgery I watched television and heard the sound of a strong heartbeat. It was the sound of my own heart. I turned the television volume down and continued to hear the sound. With every heartbeat, I heard the swooshing of blood flowing through my vessels. The sound was quite alarming. I shook my head and wondered what I was experiencing. I told Charles what I heard, and he became my doctor in that moment. However, I had an appointment with (my real doctor) Dr. Panchal the next day. So, I decided to go to bed and if I still heard it, I would tell him at my appointment.

The next morning, I woke up and I still heard the disturbing sound. It was annoying and I couldn't tune it out!

We got dressed and left for my appointment. I asked Charles to turn the music up louder as we traveled to the doctor. I closed my eyes to focus on the music in an attempt to drown out the sound in my head. It worked, thank God! When I woke up, we were pulling in the parking lot of Dr. Panchal's clinic.

The tubes that hung from my shirt made me feel a little self-conscious. I tried to conceal the tubes and the drainage bulges of my shirt by holding a towel in front of me. In the clinic, the nurse met us with a smile and complimented how well I seemed to be recovering.

While waiting, I received a call from Dr. Hunter's office. Amber, the office nurse, called with news that brought tears of joy to my heart. She excitedly reported that the pathology report showed that I was cancer free! It took all I had not to scream and leap for joy in that office, but I contained myself. I was so very thankful! I reported the good news to Charles, and he was equally thankful, and we praised the One that kept us through this process, God. I reflected on the double rainbow that I had seen before surgery. I believed it was a sign that confirmed the promises of God are yes and amen. "Yes, I was going to be fine and get through the surgery and Amen, for the clear report afterwards.

Dr. Panchal greeted us with a smile as he entered the examination room. While he removed and checked the bandaged areas, he asked a series of questions about the healing process. He was very pleased at how well the surgery site healed. I mentioned the unusual swooshing sound that I heard. He mentioned that it may have been the result of a low blood count. My iron was extremely low due to the high amount of blood I lost during the surgery. Thankfully, I didn't have to receive a blood transfusion.

It eased my mind after he shared a similar situation he experienced after having surgery. Hearing his story gave me hope, to know that even after his experience, he was alive and well. We then discussed the next phases of the reconstructive surgery process. He mentioned that before moving forward we needed to know my test results.

Undeniably, I was ecstatic to share my news of the "all clear" phone call I received. We all celebrated together in that movement. The visit ended with a scheduled follow up appointment for two weeks later.

Still feeling a little weak from surgery, I returned home and took a nap. Being sliced open and dissected like a lab frog really took a toll on my body! I couldn't move around without feeling dizzy or tired. However, I tried to be as mobile as possible, but at the same time I didn't want to push my body too hard. Around day 10 post-surgery, I felt my strength return. The swooshing sound had subsided, and I finally exhaled a sigh of relief.   An appointment was set for that afternoon with Dr. Hunter. I was ready to have the tubes removed, they were such a nuisance!

I updated Dr. Hunter regarding my visit with Dr. Panchal. She examined my incisions and stated that they were healing well. She assessed my drainage tubes and decided they should remain at least one more week. I was a little disappointed they were not removed, but thankful about the overall good report.

A week later and the drains were removed as scheduled. I almost instantly felt lighter and less pain as I moved around. Later that day, I stood in front of the mirror and examined my body closely. My breasts were gone... All that remained in their place were metal expanders, scars, tape burns, and wounds. I saw videos and read articles about some women's experiences after having their breasts removed.

Some women grieved and some considered themselves sheroes. I was now an official member of the sheroes! I was confident I'd made the best decision for me. I took charge of my health and did what needed to be done to save my life. I took an even longer gaze at myself, smiled big, and triumphantly blurted, "You did it!"

I was scheduled to return to work, but soon realized I would need more time to recover. That major surgery took a major toll on my body. I was still a little weak and had not regained the full range of motion in my arms. I wasn't back to normal just yet or even my *new normal* for that matter. Instead of returning to work in 3 weeks, I took an additional two weeks off to ensure I could return to work safely.

While I continued to recover, I reflected on life. I evaluated my marriage, my career, and most importantly myself. I thought about all the times that I put others' needs in front of my own. I gave of myself until I was empty and had nothing else to give. Well, that had to end quickly. Before breast cancer paused my life, my day to day was so rigid and routine. My weekday typically started at 5:00 AM. I performed morning duties before work, devoted eight hours a day to my career as a nurse, sacrificed more work at home through domesticated duties, then I rested for the remaining time. I repeated this routine religiously.

Even though my body performed other duties, I was so concerned with my career that it consumed my mind. I constantly thought about things that had to be done at work. So much so that it interrupted my sleep patterns. This was a struggle, to say the least. However, I had a revelation that encouraged change. It had become a stressor and not a good one. A combination of pressures of the job, my desire to excel, and situations in life had me "STRESSED OUT!" To see me, one would never know the feelings that were bottled up inside me. The tension inside me was explosive, I couldn't suppress it any longer. There was so much pressure, and the appearance of normalcy couldn't stop my internal explosion. It was inevitable.

Like so many people, I wore a mask to conceal the way I really felt. I believed I had to be everything to everybody in whatever capacity I served. I was afraid to ask for help in fear of what people would think or say. So, I became prideful because I had accomplished so many things on my own. I know now that this way of doing things is not the best practice.

In the midst of recovery, I had to fight to maintain my peace. I struggled with the decision to step down from the position as Chief Nurse. What I thought was a blessing from God, brought so much sorrow. The scripture reveals that "The blessings of God add no sorrow." That position brought so many storms, and I concluded that it may not have been the blessing I thought it was after all. I wrestled with whether I should stay or go. Given the circumstances I knew what had to be done, but I was not ready to accept it. I even prayed about it in hopes that God would show me something different… He didn't.

When we pray, most of the time we already have the blueprint in our minds. We expect God to put His stamp of approval on our plans. I quickly learned that His thoughts are not my thoughts, and His ways are not my way. God operates at such a high altitude we cannot fathom His approach. Instead of the approval, He stamps **DENIED**. We get upset with God because our request did not align with His plan. We should be confident that God always makes the right decision. He is perfect. His plan is always to prosper us and never to harm us. There is no way our finite minds can articulate a plan for ourselves that is better than The Most High. I know this for certain.

In July of 2017, Charles applied for a position at the VA hospital and was contacted for an interview. I prayed diligently for Charles to get that job. I thought about all the perks that it could bring to us. In prayer, I even threw a negotiating factor. I promised God that I would indeed step down if Charles did not get that job. Well, Charles did not get the job in spite of my bargaining plea. He submitted application after application and did not receive so much as a call back. I wondered if this was a sign that it was just not part of the plan. Nonetheless, I made the final decision to step down from being the chief nurse.

After that, I thought "OK God, What will I do now?" I thought about the previous position I held as nurse manager at the Lawton VA Clinic. It had been vacant since my resignation in October 2016. The position was posted, and candidates were selected for interviews; however, not one was chosen. Because I knew that this position remained unfilled, I toyed with the idea of returning. But I had to see how things went first. I tucked this idea away on the shelf for safe keeping.

On August 21, 2017, there was a buzz across America concerning a solar eclipse.   People across the states were caught on camera patiently awaiting this "once in a lifetime" anomaly. Charles and I were glued to our television screen in observance of the effects of the eclipse in other areas across the world. As the solar event moved closer to Oklahoma, we got super excited. We stood in our back yard and looked up to the sky to witness the most amazing natural phenomenon. With all the chaos that went on around me, that moment reminded me of the faithfulness of God. I was in complete awe of Him. So much so that I had to document this moment in my journal.

I wrote:

"WOW!! I am excited today. Truly, this is the day you made, and I will rejoice in it. Glory, Hallelujah! We serve an awesome God. I will exalt YOU! Thank you for your many blessings upon your people which at times we often forget how you bless us. Thank you for renewing our minds today. Thank you for a refreshing wind moving across this nation. We don't take it lightly."

As I journaled, I sensed an overwhelming love. I knew that I was loved by God in spite of missteps, mishaps, and mistakes. God loves us all unconditionally. His mission is for all to be saved. Because of that He gave the greatest gift He had, his only begotten son, which was the ultimate sacrifice. If He, being all mighty and sovereign, can demonstrate humility in the capacity to sacrifice his most greatest accomplishment, most prized position… How much are we willing to give? He longs to spend time with us to cleanse us, fellowship with us, and teach us His ways of perfection. He inhabits the praises of His people. It behooves us to get into a place of worship and constant communication with God. He knows the future and how to handle every aspect of it. Isn't it grand to have a friend on your side to help you with everything?

I realized through the anticipation and excitement of the solar eclipse that dark times in life are necessary. My witness to the solar eclipse included an observation from the outside and the use of protective eyewear. Then in order to capture that beautiful moment it was necessary to look up. As I mentally walked through my life's journey, I knew I needed to remain in proper positioning through prayer, utilize protective eye wear by reading the word of God, and keeping my eyes on Jesus!

The week following the eclipse, I went to my follow-up appointment with the oncologist, Dr. Garza. This was my first visit with her since the surgery. In review of my medical records, I noticed how intensely Dr. Garza was studying the results. She pulled her chair up closer to where I was and turned the computer screen for me to see. She re-explained the results of previous reports that included the invasive cancer findings. She then linked that report to the updated situation. Based on research and the minimality of the area, the double mastectomy was a proper solution, and no adjunct treatment was recommended. She pulled up an article on the computer screen to show me statistics and recommendations. I was so happy to know that I did not have to go through the chemotherapy or radiation process. My mother was not as fortunate. She had to do both treatments. I thanked the Lord that my situation was not the same. She continued to review my records and informed me that based on negative ERPR results, I was not a candidate to be prescribed other cancer related medications. She looked at me with the biggest smile and said, "You are all done and cancer free."

Such a weight was lifted off my shoulder and I felt like I could finally breathe, *again*. She discussed her plan of follow up within 6 months. Then she encouraged a follow up visit with the gynecologist to coordinate a date for my next surgery. Dr. Garza also notified that her office would be relocating. I was provided the information to transfer to the new location if I chose to do so. I was disappointed to hear she was leaving but I was willing to travel to her new office to continue my care with her. The thought of starting over with a new provider was too much. I went to schedule my next appointment and the clerk informed me someone would call me to schedule my appointment.

I was so excited to call my family and share the great news. I was cancer free, glory to God! When I recorded the day's entry in my journal, I read over an entry from my surgery day. After a four-month bout with cancer, I was cancer free. Even though there were a few other surgeries in the works, reconstructive and hysterectomy, I was happy and grateful to God that I no longer had to worry about cancer.

As the weekend neared, Charles and I made plans to visit our boys on a game day. This was my first long trip/outing since surgery. As I got dressed, I was conscious about the clothing I wore. I made sure my clothing fit loosely, I wanted to conceal my bare chest as much as possible. Most people did not know about my condition, but I was afraid of the stares, I wondered if people would notice I no longer had breasts.

We arrived early, so we sat in the truck until the game started. At Fans Day, the fans would line up, be given a schedule for the season, and walk through with the football players in hopes of getting their autograph. As we walked up to the line, I spotted Jacques and waved without lifting my arms too high. I was so excited to see him and proud to support him throughout his college endeavors. I got closer to the table, and I could see the other guys at the table looking toward me and talking with Jacques. We arrived in front of Jacques' table, and he gave me a hug. His teammates were still looking at me and all said hello. As I continued to walk around to the other tables, I saw my nephew, Devontrae. I could see his big smile three to four tables away. He also walked around the table and gave me a hug.

Both he and Jacques continued to greet the other fans with the team.

I was starting to get tired and hot, so Charles walked with me back to the truck to wait until it was finished. After the event was over, the boys came to the truck and asked how I felt. They both were amazed at how I looked. Jacques told me his friends said your mom does not look like she was sick. Charles quickly replied, "But God" and I smiled. Jacques complimented my hairstyle and how well I looked. The last time they saw me was after surgery on August 7th and trust me that was not a good look.

The day that I was rushed to the emergency room, my husband called our boys to let them know what was happening. That phone call caused a great deal of fear and anxiety and of course, they thought the worst. They shared that when they received the news, the team stopped in the middle of practice to pray for me.

My boys attended a private, Christian university in Shawnee, Oklahoma called Oklahoma Baptist University. I trusted this institution with my boys because their foundation is God and prayer. I was a first-hand witness to this with our many visits to the campus. I was grateful that my boys had people around them to pray and support them through our journey. We had dinner with the boys and headed home. It was a very long day but very rewarding and I enjoyed every moment of it!

We went to church on Sunday and enjoyed our time in service. It was nice seeing everyone, as this was my first Sunday back after having surgery. Since most people did not know, it was awkward that I did not permit hugs, but I believe they understood.

During praise and worship, I lifted my hands as high as I could despite having a few sharp pains here and there. I had so much to praise God for and I was determined to praise Him through the pain. After service, we relaxed for the rest of the day. I was exhausted from the day's activities. Each day I extended myself a little more to build my strength. I was determined to get back to a state of normalcy, but I understood that it would take some time to fully recover.

Chapter 6

Keep It Moving

When I returned to work, my supervisor placed me at a local outpatient clinic for the next few weeks. I felt a plethora of emotions when I thought about returning to work. I was nervous, scared, anxious, and self-conscious that people would stare while trying to recognize my physical differences. I put on a blouse that camouflaged my chest. My body had gone through some significant changes since the last time I graced the office with my presence. Most of the staff knew the gist of my battle, but not many knew about my mastectomy. Although I felt strange, I survived it.

Not much had changed while I was out. There were meetings after meetings that flooded my calendar daily. Since I was not onsite, Skype meetings were scheduled so I could be in attendance. My schedule permitted a half-day work period, but by 9 o'clock in the morning, I was *already* exhausted. I finished out the workday and went home for a nap. I needed to discuss my decision to step down with my supervisor, but with the days being so busy I could not find the time to do so. It was a short work week, so I decided to wait a few more days before I set up a time to meet with her.

The follow up visits went well, and I looked forward to the reconstruction process. After surgery, tissue expanders were placed under the skin in my breast area to prepare the skin for surgery. I went to my appointment with Dr. Panchal to start the filling of the expanders. I researched and read up on the procedure to prepare myself for the visit. Dr. Panchal and the nurse explained the procedure. He could tell I was nervous and told me to relax. He assessed both implants for placement and cleansed the area. As the nurse handed him the needle, I closed my eyes to try and relax. I felt a tiny stick as Dr. Panchal inserted the needle into the tiny valve under my skin. I was surprised to have feeling in that area since the rest of the breast was numb.

As he injected the solution, I felt a little pressure on both sides, but it was fine. He told me it was necessary to return for appointments to fill the expanders. I had to determine if I would come every week or every other week. The reconstructive surgery had already been finalized for December 26, 2017. That was the first appointment Charles did not accompany me, I felt like I was walking a green mile.

I felt sad, as to why he did not come with me. Was my illness starting to be too much for him?

I told Charles about my appointment but never mentioned how I felt. I did not believe I needed any help, but in these moments, I realized I needed the comfort of my support system. Later that afternoon, I experienced tightness in my chest. Dr. Panchal did mention that there would be discomfort with each fill of the expanders. So, I didn't worry, I just popped two Tylenol and went about my day.

When I finally decided to inform my supervisor of my decision to step down, I scheduled our meeting via telephone for the end of the day. She called and we talked about work matters and how my recovery was going. Prior to our meeting, I experienced quite a few workdays that were beyond stressful, and I broke down into an uncontrollable sobbing. At the time, it was necessary for me to take control of my health by ensuring I did everything I could to heal properly.

My supervisor told me, "You have a lot going on right now. Take some time to think about this more." I knew today was the day and I was confident in the decision. My voice trembled as I skirted around the purpose of the meeting. I finally mustered up enough courage to say, "After much thought and consideration, I have decided to step down and return to my previous job." There was a brief silence on the phone. My supervisor then asked a few questions but ultimately accepted my decision. I was blessed to have developed such a good working relationship with her.

When she first arrived at our organization, I was terrified at the idea of a new supervisor. However, I listened to her and followed her vision for us. I felt more comfortable around her and respected her as my new leader. My supervisor arrived at our organization during a very unsettling time. Our current nursing leadership team had suddenly switched up within a 90-day process. People resigned and retired unexpectedly and left us unsure of the fate and future of our jobs. I later learned that after I shared my decision with my supervisor, she went to the Director of Medical Center, so upset that he thought the cancer was worse than reported. I continued to work in the position for another month.

At times, I regretted my decision and wanted to stay. One day I received a text from one of my nurses. She asked how I was doing and told me she was thinking of me. As I continued to read, she revealed that she prayed for me and reminded me not to forget what I promised God. When I saw that, I knew what it meant, and I knew what I had to do. I needed to put my request to step down in writing and forward it to my supervisor.

It was the end of the day, on a Friday when I finally submitted the formal request to step down as chief nurse and return to nurse manager. As I drove home, I was torn about the email. I told myself, "It was the best thing to do." I continued in the role for another two weeks before I officially stepped down on October 15, 2017. I worked closely with my supervisor to find a replacement and allow for proper training for the new chief nurse. My colleagues were very supportive of my decision, and this made stepping down a little easier. I told the Nurse Managers my decision to step down and they were very supportive of my decision.

On the following Thursday, the staff surprised me with a farewell breakfast. I was so overwhelmed with joy from their kind gestures. While sitting at a table with the staff, one of the nurses shared how my farewell speech touched her. She herself had struggled with a decision concerning her job and family. Hearing my story helped her to solidify the decision she had to make. The more I shared my journey with people, the more I learned that this was not about me. In fact, it was so much bigger. The journey prepared me to encourage others in their time of need. I truly believe that until you have experienced certain things it is nearly impossible to fully understand how to help others.

One Sunday I heard my Pastor say, "You do not know God as your healer until He has healed you." I have heard that saying many times. But on that particular day, it hit differently. I did not know at that moment what was ahead of me, but today, I understand. I can truly say that God is my healer. I am not just quoting the scripture, but I am a living testimony, a walking epistle that God is a healer, and His word will not and cannot return void.

It was a bittersweet moment when I packed my office. However, I knew that the change was necessary, and I had to trust God along the way. I returned to the Lawton VA Clinic as a nurse manager the following Monday. The staff welcomed me back with open arms. Having to adjust to a new normal was a heck of a process. The team that once knew me in the capacity as chief nurse reclaimed me as a peer. I don't think that adjustment was nearly as hard for them as it was for me but thank God for humility. That was a time I had to hand over complete control to God because I faced the most challenges in the workplace.

My work was criticized, I was ridiculed and talked about, half the time people would forget my name. Oftentimes, I resorted to my office to take a cry break. I felt like I had made the worst decision of my life and I wanted to give up on that disaster of a career. I hated going to work. I wanted to escape all those feelings by giving it all up and never looking back.

I became overwhelmed AGAIN with the decisions to move forward in the next phases after my health crisis. I had recurring visits with Dr. Panchal every two to three weeks for expander fills. The hysterectomy was still in progress and the date was set for November 15, 2017. Recovery time was approximately six weeks, and I did not want to be out of work again for such a long period of time. I made a request to my supervisor to consider approval for Telework for a few weeks during my recovery time. Initially, my doctor did not agree to the suggested Telework, but later changed his mind if I agreed to take the full six weeks before returning to work.

As my surgery date neared, I arranged coverage for my clinic while I was out. It was the end of the rating period for yearly staff appraisals, and they had to be complete before I left. It was a challenge, but I was able to get everything submitted by the deadline.

The day of surgery came, and Charles and I went to the hospital. This was surgery number three at this particular hospital, number four overall. By now I was so familiar with the process, I could pretty much conduct it all by myself. After the intake process was completed, Dr. Meza explained the ins and outs of the surgery including possible complications of death. At that point, I completely lost it. I was terrified. That was my fourth surgery over the span of a year, and I did not know how much more slicing and dicing my body could take. Apparently, Charles shared the same feelings because he cried too.

"I am tired." I said exhaustively, "I just want all of this to be over." The nurse handed me a Kleenex to wipe my eyes. I felt bad for crying in front of everyone, but I needed to release those emotions.

I waited for about an hour before the nurse came to take me to the operating room. Charles kissed me and said, "I love you," as they rolled me away. While the nurses strapped me to the table, I heard them talking. The anesthesiologist gave the medication through an IV push, then just like magic I awakened in recovery. The room was dimly lit and cold. First thing I did was thank God for bringing me through yet another surgery.

I became a regular at this hospital. Some of the same staff that cared for me through previous surgeries cared for me again. The surgery was successful and now I was on the road to recovery once again. I was connected to a PCA pump to administer pain medication to manage my pain levels. The nurse informed me that I was prescribed morphine to ease my pain. She gave instructions on how to self-administer and asked if I had any questions. I did have one question, one silent question. I have a very high pain tolerance, and I wanted to know why in the world Dr. Meza prescribed morphine for pain management. A little while later, I found out why.

It was dinner time, and I was hungry. However, my body could only tolerate clear liquids. Charles was quite considerate, and he refused to eat in front of me. So, he left the room to have his Chinese food. A few hours later, I felt an increasing amount of pain in my abdominal region. I pushed the button that released medication into my IV, but it did not help. So, I turned on my side in an attempt to get comfortable, but the pain got worse. The nurse in pre-op told me to make sure they gave me something for gas. When I requested medicine for gas, it was denied because none had been ordered.

The nurse advised me to lie on my left side to relieve some of the pain. I looked at her then looked at my arm, with all the IV tubing and wires running from it and I thought to myself, "This lady can't be serious." The pain persisted for a while, but I fought through it. I tried to sleep but the constant in and out traffic from the staff kept that from happening. I looked over at Charles all snuggled and relaxed in that chair and grumbled, "At least one of us is able to rest."

The next morning, Dr. Meza made his rounds early and signed my papers for discharge. He later told me he was truly concerned when I cried before my surgery. He visited me at least three times while I was in the hospital. I told him I appreciated him giving me the special attention because I needed it. While waiting to be discharged, a student nurse was assigned to care for me. She came in to do her assessment with the instructor. This reminded me of my clinical days as a student nurse. I was scared to death that I was going to hurt the patients. I could see the fear in her eyes as she carefully disconnected me from the machines and assisted me to the restroom.

That was my first time up after surgery. The doctors instructed me to stay overnight so they could ensure I didn't have any bladder issues. Thankfully, I was able to use the bathroom after they removed the Foley catheter without any problems, and I was discharged.

The ride home was a little uncomfortable. Every little bump and hump in the road caused me pain. Though the road was rough, literally, we made it safely. Later that afternoon, I received a call from the hospital informing us that flowers had been sent to me, it was the nursing staff at my job. I thought it was so sweet and I was so appreciative of their kindness. Charles went back to the hospital to get my flowers and we rested for the rest of the night.

I felt stronger as the days went by. Thanksgiving was less than a week away, so we prepared our grocery list. Our menu included all the side fixings and desserts. This particular year we had to do things a little differently… I was still in recovery mode from the surgery. However, I was adamant about cooking! Our boys were home from college, and they assisted me with the prep for our favorite dishes. I knew if I did not make the sweet potato pies and candied yams, the boys would be disappointed.

The sweet potato pies are my mom's recipe. Every time I make them, I am reminded of the last time my mother and I made sweet potato pies and sour cream pound cake together. That memory gave me the push I needed to get past the exhaustion I felt, and the desserts came out perfectly. We had a deliciously unforgettable Thanksgiving dinner and that year we truly had so much to be thankful for. The laughter, love, and liveliness my family and I shared were priceless and irreplaceable.

A few days later, my oldest granddaughter, Alicia was scheduled to have surgery. I wanted to be there with her and my son, but I could not travel, I was still recovering. We Facetimed before and after her surgery and I thanked God that everything went according to plan.

My follow up appointment with Dr. Meza and final pathology reports were finally in. The results revealed NO cancer! However, he did give a report of endometriosis and scar tissue in my uterus. This explained the painful and heavy menstruation cycles I had. In spite of that, all was well. I was healing and getting stronger every day.

I was so glad I didn't have all three surgeries at one time. It was too much for my body to handle all at once. I was unable to use the upper part of my body after the double mastectomy and the lower part of my body after the hysterectomy. It would have been way too much for the both of us. I thank God for wisdom.

Chapter 7

Coming to Terms with Myself

I sat in my recliner and listened to a church message on YouTube, I thought to myself, "Oh my goodness, half of my lady parts are gone!" I cried as I pondered everything I'd been through that year. How one diagnosis caused a snowball effect of unfortunate health events. I felt a feeling of anger arise that had to be tamed quickly. Then I heard the Lord say, "But you still have your spirit." After I heard this, I wrote this in my journal:

"Through it all, I shield your spirit. In times of distress, and when you feel like everything that makes you a female is gone, remember my - I am your shield. We are connected in SPIRIT, not by your breast, uterus, fallopian tubes, or ovaries. I created every inch of you before you were formed in your mother's womb and our connection is much greater than organs and parts of your physical body. I stand tall as a refuge, shielding everything that tries to come against your spirit to turn you away from me. No weapon formed against you will prosper my daughter. I am your God and I hide you under my mighty wings. You are shielded for life!"

The greatest gift I happily accepted during my journey was the time I spent with God. I longed to be in the presence of God so I could hear what He spoke to me. My relationship with God deepened and I needed that more than anything!

I finally finished the last fill for the expanders. I was happy when Dr. Panchal said, "this is it for now." I had four weeks before I would have surgery to have the implants inserted. The expanders were getting a little more uncomfortable with each fill. I was still extremely body conscious, so I wore clothes that did not draw attention to my chest area.

A few weeks later Charles and I attended a Christmas Comedy Party in our community. I brought a beautiful red and black gown and was so excited to wear it. The gown fit perfectly. I looked in the mirror at myself and saw pure beauty. I took pictures with Charles to capture the moment and I shared a few snaps with family and friends. I felt beautiful and at that moment I was not concerned about being breastless. Undeniably, I am a phenomenal woman, and I looked the part.

We saw several of our friends and had a great time! I received so many compliments and I spread my feathers and strutted my stuff just a little bit prouder. Charles and I needed that time of laughter after so many hard days. We usually traveled home to Florida for Christmas but that year we could not. My very last surgery was scheduled for the day after Christmas.

I love decorating during the Christmas season. I love filling each room with the sights and sounds of Christmas. We enjoyed a quiet Christmas that year. I was nervous about my surgery the next day but tried to enjoy the day with the family. We made plans to stay overnight in a hotel after the surgery in case of an emergency. I had surgery at the Surgery Center in Oklahoma City, OK, which is an hour and half from our house. Later that evening, my throat began to feel scratchy. I did not think much of it and went to bed. When I woke up the next morning, it was better but still there. We drove to Oklahoma City for the surgery. The boys were asleep in the back of the truck, and I closed my eyes most of the trip but could not fall asleep. I wasn't feeling the best, and my nerves were getting the best of me.

We arrived at the Surgery Center early. So, I checked in with the clerk while Charles and the boys got some breakfast. The waiting room was already filled with other patients and their loved ones. I thought it would be a slow day because it was the day after Christmas. Surprisingly, it was not!

This would be my fifth surgery! Once again, I found myself naked and afraid lying on a cutting board. My throat *still* felt scratchy, and it seemed to be getting worse. When I told the nurse and doctor, they did not seem the least bit concerned. It was time to go to the operating room. My heart was beating rapidly as the nurses strapped me to the table and connected me to the monitors. The anesthesiologist asked me if I was nervous. I quickly admitted I was. In an assured tone, he said, "This one is simple. It's nothing like the last time you were here, OK. Try to relax."

The procedure I had is known as "the swap." My tissue expanders were removed and replaced with breast implants. Dr. Panchal and I discussed my desired cup size for my implants. Prior to my surgery, the nurse measured my chest. I was shocked to learn I was a D cup! I had been wearing the wrong bra size for a while. However, I was quite firm when I told Dr. Panchal not to oversize my implants.

The anesthesiologist sedated me and when I woke up, I was in the recovery area. I was in pain, so the nurse gave me some medication. She informed me that my surgery was successful and that I'd be discharged after a few hours of observation. My chest was tightly secured in white bandages. When I got dressed, I put on my bra to securely hold everything in place. I'd made the mistake of not securing my chest after the double mastectomy and the pain was unforgettably excruciating. I vowed not to make that mistake again!

I was packed and ready to go. My discharge papers were signed and off we went. Oklahoma's weather was a little chilly that day and I'd forgotten to pack a coat. I had on a sweater, but the piercing wind cut through my sweater like a hot knife through butter. The nurse gave me a blanket for reinforcement. As we made our way to the hotel, we noticed snow flurries were falling. Although, it was a beautiful sight… I didn't want to be caught in it. I couldn't wait to get to the warmth of the hotel and have a good night's rest.

I woke up the next morning feeling strong and refreshed. I glanced over my bandaged chest, and I saw that my implants were much smaller than the expanders. During the follow-up for my dressing removal, I told the doctor the implants were smaller than I anticipated. He chuckled and matter-of-factly said, "We can always go larger!" I quickly responded, "NO!"

I was truly blessed to have such great doctors to care for me during my journey. They listened to me, they cried with me, and they prayed with and for me. When I walked through my mother's breast cancer journey, I constantly reminded her doctors and nurses to provide excellent care. Quite often my mom said, "Don't say anything because I don't know how they'll treat me if you're not here!" As a healthcare professional, I was furious with the lack of compassion some of the nurses had for my mother and other patients, so I spoke up as her advocate. It was my duty to ensure my mother and others were given quality health care.

Side Note: Always be an advocate for your health and your family members. I hate to admit this, but everyone who works within

When I woke up the next morning, my throat was hurting. The pain intensified when I swallowed. I couldn't eat because it was too painful. I was surprised at the pain in my throat. I expected the pain to be in my chest, but *this* was different. I rested throughout the day, and I drank as much as I could to stay hydrated.

Around 6:00 pm, I awakened with chills. I went into the living room and asked Charles to take my temperature. It was 102.1 degrees. I was scared and I didn't know what was going on. I had just seen Dr. Panchal the previous day. "Oh no, not again." My mind went back to that day in August when I was rushed to the emergency room 24 hours after surgery. I decided to just take some Tylenol and go to bed.

After a few hours, my temperature broke and I felt a little better. I tried to eat some soup, but my throat was *still* extremely sore. Later that night, I checked my temperature, and I had a fever of 102.6. I told Charles I needed to go to the emergency room immediately!

When we arrived at the ER the nurses immediately screened me and took me to the back. Then the doctor came in and assessed me. I told him I'd recently had surgery and the name of my doctor. After he left, the nurse made a snide comment about getting breast implants. I told her, "I had breast cancer and that is why I have implants, not because I want bigger boobs." Her insensitivity upset me, and I wanted to say more… but I didn't. Although she apologized, I did not want her caring for me anymore.

The doctor ordered a major workup that included blood work and x-rays. He contacted Dr. Panchal and discussed my case with him. Dr. Panchal told him to check me for the flu. The nurse came in and took a swab to test for the flu. As the doctor shared my test results, my blood count was within range, and he was unsure as to why I had such a high fever. He planned to send me home on antibiotics and instructed me to follow up with Dr. Panchal. I was already on antibiotics from Dr. Panchal, now this doctor wanted to change to something different.

I asked the doctor for the result of the flu swab. He did not have my results and looked slightly surprised when I asked him about it. He left my room to retrieve the results.

When he returned and told me I had a positive reading for the flu. I felt a little better knowing the cause of my fever. The doctor asked if I received the flu vaccine and I replied, "Yes." He gave me a care-guide for the flu and told me to follow up with Dr. Panchal. I was finally being discharged *again.*

I had an appointment with Dr. Hunter in a few hours. So, I put my mask on and headed to the appointment. Dr. Hunter assessed my chest area around the implants and said I was healing well. I told her I was in the ER the night before and was diagnosed with the flu. She told me to stay away from others, drink plenty of fluids and rest. I was scheduled to see her in a month.

Charles and I returned home, and I went to bed. We decided it was best if he slept in another room, so he would not get sick. Charles and the boys cared for me over the next few days. It was funny to see them come in the room with their masks on to bring me food and drinks. I could hear them in the other room talking and laughing but I was so weak and could barely stay awake. I was so sick from the flu; I don't even remember the recovery from my surgery.

Sunday, December 31, 2017, Charles and the boys went to church, and I was still running a fever, so I was unable to attend. I mustered up enough strength to walk to the living room and sit on the sofa, while they were gone. I opened my iPad to Bishop T. D. Jakes, Sunday service. I listened to praise and worship and the message. It was New Year's Eve, so he encouraged everyone to join their New Year's Eve service later that evening.

The message was titled, "Get over yourself." The scripture reference was Ruth 1: 1-15. I heard the story of Ruth many times, but that day Bishop Jakes presented it in a whole new way. He spoke more about Naomi and how she contributed to the story of Ruth. The message made me realize it was time for me to pass the baton to those around me. I thought of my experiences and how I needed to share with other women who maybe struggling or feeling hopeless. So many topics came to mind as I listened to the message. At that moment, I began to praise and worship God. I felt my fever break, and as I walked around the living room, I felt myself getting stronger. The message gave me hope I needed to look forward to the year of 2018.

The year 2017, shook me to my core. By December 2017, I realized that I had to "Get over myself," if I wanted to keep moving forward into what God had for me and my family. When I started this journey in April 2017, I did not know if tomorrow was promised… and I still don't know. Thankfully, I understand what I went through was necessary. My life didn't end but it changed *for the better.* I was glad to be alive and cancer free. When I faced the possibility of death so closely, my gratitude for life, health, and strength increased *divinely.*

Chapter 8

What's Next?

It was the New Year, and I had one more week of recovery before I returned to work. I had recurring doctor appointments every three months to six months. I promised myself that I would take better care of myself by limiting the stress in my life. The long hours at work, taking on multiple assignments, and being concerned with other people's problems were no longer a priority for me.

For years, I spent much of my life reviewing the past and projecting the future… I neglected to live my life in the present. I tried to wish away things in my past while trying to rush the future. Sadly, that left no time for the present. Today, I am intentional about living in the present. I cherish every moment of every day.

A friend once told me, "Treat every day as your birthday." Since then, I have learned to celebrate life daily. The loss of my mother and other family members to cancer coupled with my battle with the brutal disease was enough to drive me insane. However, I am here today by the grace of God. Many days I wanted to give up and throw in the towel, but I held on to hope and the promises of God to see things through.

With the progression of 2018, I learned so much [more] myself and what I needed to do to maximize my potential. My body and mind had changed so much that I was no longer the same person. I was more in tune with my mind, my body, and my soul. To this day, I fight to keep my mind free of negativity and unproductive thoughts. After the course of treatment has come to completion for patients with cancer, the doctors continue routine schedule checks to monitor conditions. That in itself is stressful. It can be a time of celebration as the cancer is in remission, but it can also create angst at the thought of cancer recurring.

April 28, 2018, approximately one year after my initial diagnosis, I celebrated a cancer free milestone. I wanted to travel to Mount Scott, a prominent mountain located northwest of Lawton, Oklahoma. It was perfect for reflecting. On that bright and sunny Saturday, Charles and I drove up the mountain. As we got closer to the top, we saw cars were parked alongside the road. There were several visitors on the mountain, but I was determined to find the perfect reflective spot and capture that moment in time.

I wore an orange shirt with the words Grateful, Thankful and Blessed printed on the front. As I looked out over the land, I cried tears of joy, happiness, and relief. I was so thankful that I made it through one of the hardest trials of my life and I'm alive to tell my story. I live a FULL life with no restrictions. I was afraid of heights, so the trip up the mountain not only symbolized a victory after a perceived defeat, but it also represented a conquered fear.

A month later, I visited my eldest son, Cedric, and his family in North Carolina. That was the first time we had a face-to-face visit in person in a year. Charles, the boys, and I flew to visit over the Memorial Day holiday. When we arrived at the airport, we were excited and full of anticipation. When I walked up to my son's car, my granddaughter's face lit up after she saw me. It was priceless. She screamed, "Nana", and jumped out of the car seat and gave me the biggest hug.

I was not able to pick her up but to embrace her in my arms was such a joy. I didn't see my son; he must have gone through another door to enter the airport. When I turned around to look for him, he came up behind me wearing the biggest smile ever. He embraced me with a long, warm, and loving hug. We were all together once again and my heart was full of love, joy, and happiness. As I looked into the faces of my dear loved ones, I smiled and reminded myself that my fight was for me and them. We won together! For this very reason I kept and will continue to keep hope alive.

In October 2018, I participated in my first Spirit of Survival Race. That race was a big fundraising event to raise money for cancer research for the local cancer centers in Southwest Oklahoma. I encouraged my family and women from my local church to participate in the event. I have always had a passion to promote breast cancer awareness. Each year at our church, I lead events with our Health Ministry for breast cancer awareness. I am thankful to my Pastors for allowing us to share preventive health tips with the church congregations.

In response to church participation in the Spirit of Survival Race, our women's group ordered t-shirts stamped with the phrase "Team Henderson - For some it is more than a race..." I was presented with the task of participating in the 5K event and I graciously accepted. Many of my supporters teamed up to walk with me. The support was overwhelming, and I cannot fully express my appreciation to those who supported me through my entire journey.

I finished the race by running across the finish line with a huge, Kool-Aid smile spread across my face. Although my cancer journey was a tough one, there were many benefits that I reaped because of it. My son, Cedric, was an Army Instructor at North Carolina State University during that time. He collaborated with the sports department at the school, and he had the entire volleyball team dress out in matching t-shirts to honor breast cancer survivors.

In addition, I was selected to attend the Play4Kay basketball game at North Carolina State University. The Play4Kay is a large fundraising initiative to unite players, coaches, officials, and fans to support a greater cause. The Play4Kay event was set up in honor of Coach Sandra Yow, who succumbed to cancer and passed away in 2009 after a lengthy 22-year, on-again, off-again battle with the disease.

In February 2019, I flew to Raleigh, North Carolina, and led the 0-2 years group of breast cancer survivors onto the basketball center court. There were hundreds of people, ranging to 35+ years as a breast cancer survivor. The gym was filled with fans and families dressed in pink to celebrate and honor the survivors and donate to the cause. Prior to the game, my son arranged a family photo shoot. When I look back over the photos we took, I remember the love, joy, and support. It felt more than good to give back, I was fulfilling and purposeful. The event was televised live on ESPN. Our family and friends were reminded to watch the game and to look for me during the halftime show.

The time came to prepare for the halftime show. Cedric escorted me to my assigned area. I met with the coordinator of our group, and she gave me a big sign to hold high as we entered onto the court. A flood of ladies joined us as we gathered around each other and exchanged names and stories. Everyone was excited and nervous at the same time. One lady shared that she was cancer free for only three weeks but wanted so badly to be part of this great event. I told her that she could stick with me. As we lined up and moved closer to the starting point, she held my arm firmly.

Our group was the first group to enter the court, so I had to make sure to get the coordinates right. There was a cord on the floor, and we had to be careful not to trip over it. The announcer gave the introduction and called the 0–2-year group. I went onto the court with my sign held high as I led our group of beautiful survivors.

Everyone gave a standing ovation as we entered the basketball arena. We all met half court, smiling and cheering each other on. There were television cameras everywhere, it was so exciting. Afterwards, I received texts and pictures from family members that spotted me and captured the moment, it was a beautiful feeling.

Each survivor had their own unique story. I met one woman that had been cancer-free for 25 years. I can and will use her victory as a reminder that if God did it for her, He can do it for me *too*. In that moment, we were all united as we celebrated each other. We knew that our story was not everyone's story. Many did not survive their battle with cancer, and we also honored those we lost. If I never have an opportunity like that again, that night will forever be a part of my I- Survived legacy.

I met some amazingly resourceful women. They shared information through organized support groups and provided educational resources. They inspired me to reach out to more women. I could not find a support group that coordinated with my work schedule when I needed it. The support I received came from a group of survivor friends that reached out to encourage me. I still struggle to find a support group that has flexible hours.

In my attempt to offer support to others, I also use my independent business credentials to donate H.O.P.E. Care Packages to our local Cancer center. The packages include a regimen of skin care products for patients. I am honored to be in a position to help and bless others. I have and will continue to do what God has called me to do.

July 29, 2019, I celebrated my 50th birthday with my family and friends [at home] in White Springs, FL. They traveled from near and far to celebrate with me. After the good time we had our family reunion, I told Charles I wanted to recreate that feeling of family for my 50th birthday. That request was honored, and we had an amazing time. My boys gave their toasts and honored me as they expressed their admiration of my strength and fortitude during my journey.

Their heartfelt words brought tears to my eyes and reminded me how blessed I was.

When I received my diagnosis, I wasn't sure if I would see my forty eighth birthday let alone my fiftieth. The night was full of laughter, feasting, dancing, and celebrating life. I danced until my feet hurt. I enjoyed every moment of that night and I felt like the queen of the night. My father-in-law attended the party. We shared a beautiful dance! Little did I know, our first dance would also be our last...

In September of 2019 my father-in-law passed away. His death was so unexpected and took our family by surprise. Before his death, a close friend of mine as well as my uncle had gotten reports that their cancer had returned. I was terrified of cancer returning to my body. My emotions were all over the place and I felt like screaming.

Faith & Therapy

I had an appointment with my PCP and during the screening with the nurse, I broke down crying. Every question she asked me during the depression screening I scored positive. I noticed the nurse was rushing with the questions at the end and immediately left the room. Mrs.

Bowman entered the room and asked, "How are you doing?" I cried profusely as I attempted to tell her the reason for the visit. I finally just blurted out, "I need help!" I told her about my uncle, father-in-law, and close friend. Mrs. Bowman was the one who gave me my test results of breast cancer. She was very familiar with every part of my journey. It seemed as though I fell into a depression and needed additional help outside of what my family, friends, and supporters could offer. Mrs. Bowman submitted a request for a consultation with a mental health provider.

Yes, I went to therapy, and I still attend sessions as needed. Counseling opened up a whole new world of feelings and emotions I didn't know existed. My bout with cancer and the fear of recurrence brought me there, but I soon discovered that I had a history of significant emotional losses, hurts, and traumas that were never grieved properly. Counseling has taught me more about myself. Just as I advocate for preventive screenings, I am also an advocate for addressing and assessing mental health. Don't be ashamed to admit you need help. I still get emotional when I tell my story and talk about my mom and others I have lost.

However, I understand that it is ok and the more I share, the stronger I will get.

I was invited to a breast cancer awareness celebration for survivors in October 2019. It was great to dress up in pink and celebrate with the other survivors. We were given the opportunity to share our stories. It took the ladies and me a few minutes to decide who would go first. As the first survivor spoke and others continued, I debated whether or not I would share my story. The difference between those ladies and myself was that they had all been through chemotherapy and radiation, I had not. Those ladies were the real heroes with all they had been through. I was the last one left to speak. All the attention fell on me as everyone waited with anticipation to hear what I had to say. My decision to share was made in that very instant.

The lady standing next to me held my hand as I told my story. We all appreciated and commended one another for having the courage and strength to share. Fear attempted to surface, but I did not allow it to silently paralyze me. I will continue to speak out to help encourage others. We were given a gift for our participation. My gift was a pretty pink butterfly. I keep it on my dresser to remind me that I have gone through a metamorphosis. Now, it's time to shed the cocoon and spread my beautiful wings and fly.

After experiencing the best of what life could be, it seemed short lived when the not so good news started to roll in. First, I received a letter in the mail in reference to a recall on breast implants. I vaguely heard something on the news about that, but I verified the type that I had and dismissed it because at that time it didn't apply to me… or so I thought.

Then, we received a phone call about my Uncle Howard weeks before Thanksgiving. They reported that his health was failing fast and eventually he was placed into Hospice.

Happy Thanksgiving! On this day we gathered with family face to face or and virtually. We Facetimed our uncles and other family members. Charles, the boys, and I had a very Happy Thanksgiving.

The boys prepared for their upcoming college graduation. We were excited for all that they were able to accomplish. These times are bittersweet for a parent. It's the end of one era and the beginning of another. As a parent we want our kids to experience all success with minimal to no hardships. We want the very best for our kids, but we know life is unpredictable. At this point we are charged with the most difficult task… letting go.

Graduation day finally arrived, and we were super excited. Two of my brothers traveled to Oklahoma to attend their graduation. Our sons faced so much adversity during their college years, but we are thankful that they were determined and finished strong. This day was all about the boys; Charles and I couldn't have felt more proud than we did in that moment! God gave us three young men to mold, shape, teach, and assist them in navigating life's courses. There is only so far that we could take them. However, we thank God, they made it this far.

At the start of the ceremony, we received a phone notification that our uncle had passed away. I was torn between feelings. I wanted to cry but this moment was just too joyous and exciting to let sadness be the dominant emotion. The graduation concluded and everyone gathered for photos. I had to decide whether or not to share the news of my uncle's passing. The family needed to know, but I did not want to put a damper on the mood.

At the post celebration dinner, I decided that they should know so I shared the news. I called everyone together and we stood in a circle, I informed them of our uncle's passing then followed with encouragement to continue in celebration.

Two days later another family member passed away unexpectedly. Charles and I traveled to Florida the day after Christmas to attend both funerals. We arrived back home on New Year's Eve to celebrate with our boys. While traveling back home, Jacques called and shared that he got the job he applied for. It was great to hear some good news and know that God was still answering our prayers.

We welcomed in a new year 2020 as a family in church as we usually do. None of us knew what the year of 2020 would be but we all greatly anticipated an exciting year. Charles and I got Jacques settled in his new apartment and ready for his new job. Our nephew was still looking for employment and spent most of the year with us, until he started his new job in June 2020.

We all stood together as we faced the COVID 19 pandemic. With so much uncertainty in the world around us, we held tightly to the Word of God and prayer. In August of 2020, I went to the doctor for a complaint of shoulder pain, which led to him sending me for x-rays. I worked in the building with my PCP, and he sent me a message on skype with the results of my x-ray. I did not think anything major was wrong and knew it was protocol to get updated x-rays before sending the patient to the Chiropractor.

In the message, the doctor said my shoulder was good but there was an area on my lung, and I needed to get a chest CT scan done. I replied and asked if I could come to his office. My heart was pounding, and my mind went straight to oh my god, do I have cancer. I went to his office to talk with him. I was crying and pacing back and forth. He explained the report and tried to reassure me not to jump to the worst-case scenario.

I left his office, grabbed my phone, and called Charles. As I walked outside of the clinic, I told him what the doctor said. He encouraged me to calm down and told me he was on his way to the clinic. I went to my truck and waited for Charles. I was scared and was not expecting to hear that news from the doctor. I had applied for a job in Austin, TX right before this and was selected for the position.

As I sat waiting on Charles, it felt like April 2017 was happening all over again. Charles arrived and we talked about the results. He prayed with me and assured me that I was going to be alright. It was almost time for me to get off, so I went back to the office to gather my things and met him at home. I had a counseling session via telephone that evening with my counselor. I was so devastated by the news that I could not make it through the whole session. I was so afraid and did not know if I could go through another diagnosis of cancer.

The appointment for the CT-scan was scheduled quickly. I went to the appointment and waited a few days for the results. Dr. Lopez came to my office a few days later to give me the results. The scan showed scar tissue possibly from a previous infection or inflammation. I was so relieved. I was told I'd be screened again at three months and nine months. My three-month report showed no change. As I write this book, I am awaiting the results at the nine month follow up.

As fall approached, I became excited about upcoming events for breast cancer awareness in October. The COVID pandemic, caused several events to be canceled or to be done virtually. I signed up to support the Mary Kay Foundation 5K Virtual Race. Charles and the boys joined me as we walked around our neighborhood and shared each mile on Facebook Live. I had several family and friends donate to the Foundation during this event.

One morning during my prayer time, I asked God to give me guidance on how to grow my Mary Kay business. The devotion I read that morning was from Psalm 46:10, "Be still and know that I am God: I will be exalted among the heathen, I will be exalted in the earth." The practical part was to sit still for five minutes and write down that experience. I read the scripture and for five minutes, I sat still and fought to keep my thoughts from wondering.

After the timer went off, I wrote down what I heard in the stillness of the morning. I wrote my plan to start a platform for women to come together and share their stories in a safe space while celebrating each other. I wrote the name Trisha's Tea Time and the names of the ladies I needed to contact; they were breast cancer survivors and I wanted to provide space for them to share their journey and encourage other women. It amazed me how clearly my vision unfolded. I heard from God during my journey, and I knew my story would open doors for a platform to help others. All the ladies I contacted agreed to be a part of the event. Everything was coming together. The event would be aired on Zoom and Facebook live. Everyone I told about the event was excited for me and very encouraging.

I launched Trisha's Tea Time on October 31, 2020. It was a great success. I received so many calls and texts from people near and far. They complimented me on the event and expressed how much it blessed them. I sat at the dining room table when the Zoom ended and cried like a baby. I was so proud of myself for conquering fear and stepping out on faith to launch what was within me. I still conduct Trisha's Tea Time with topics given to me during my prayer time. If you need to give birth and launch *your vision* to help others… I encourage you to just do it! Everyone may not support your vision but if you believe God told you to do it, trust Him and walk in faith.

I had a speaking assignment at my church in November of 2020. Our theme was KICK Hard and Finish Strong, and my assignment was the letter "C." One point I shared with the congregation was to commit to Call. I shared how before the track runner goes to a track meet, the coach has already sent the list of runners who will compete in each event. When it is time to compete, the track runner must go to the table to check in. I ran track in high school and my boys ran track in high school and college, so I know a little about the process. The announcer makes three calls before the race, so the runners can check in. If a runner does not check in, they cannot run in that race.

I realized, if I never checked in, I would not be here today, writing, to share my story with others. My team needed me, and God needed me to check-in because He already knew the plans for my life.

What race have you failed to compete in because you felt hopeless?

Every day I decide to check in - I choose to do this through prayer, praise and worship, and keeping my HOPE alive! If you think you cannot make it, or that you are not good enough… Remember, if you commit to the call and check in, God will provide everything you need to finish strong.

Through this journey I learned how to trust God even when I could not trace Him. In order for my faith to increase, I had to take a knee and go to God in prayer. When there was chaos around me, I found a quiet place to settle myself so I could hear God speaking. I released my cares to God. This allowed me to reach for God in my time of need. I had to undergird myself with the Word of God. It gave me strength to hold on and keep fighting for my faith. Romans 10:17 states, *"Faith comes by hearing and hearing by the Word of God."* I submitted my way and will to the Lord. I had a plan, but I realized I had to go to *The Planner* and follow His plan if I was going to see this turn for my good.

I pray my journey inspires someone. Whether you are faced with a cancer diagnosis, career failure, divorced, or the loss of loved ones, there is hope and beauty on the other side. One of my favorite songs says, This joy that I have, the *world did not give it to me, and the world can't take it away. I stand on Jeremiah 29:11, "For I know the thoughts that I think toward you, says the Lord, thoughts of peace and not of evil, to give you a future and a hope."* I don't know what tomorrow may bring but I do know God has given me a future and a hope. Therefore, it is my responsibility to keep HOPE alive during every midnight hour because I'm confident that I will see the salvation of the Lord!

Final Thoughts

Hope is the feeling of wanting something to happen and believing it will; this is necessary as we face life uncertainties. My hope strengthened me and helped me endure hardships. With hope, I overcame fear, anxiety, depression, and every negative emotion that attempted to shake my faith. Hope moved me from fear to faith!

At times, hoping hurts… but we must keep hope alive because it lives in every breath and step, we take. The trials and tribulations we endure are designed to produce perseverance, character, and hope. As a walking billboard of faith, my life is a testament of God's tender mercy towards me. So, I'm committed - especially *"In the Midnight Hour to Keep H.O.P.E. Alive!"* I pray every reader makes this commitment too, so you can walk into the *BIGGER* plan God has for you!

About the Author

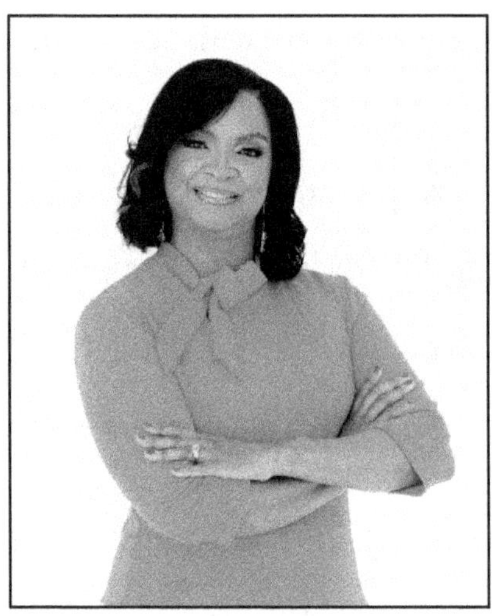

Patricia Henderson is a Registered Nurse, Licensed Ordained Minister, Entrepreneur, Breast Cancer Survivor, Veteran, and now an Author. Patricia has dedicated more than half her life to providing compassionate healthcare to her patients, family, and friends.

Patricia is the founder of Trisha's Tea Time, a community she created to give women a safe space to share their stories and encourage others. As a natural advocate for others, "Tricia" understands the importance of genuinely caring. She also leads the Health Ministry at her local church, and she helps coordinate events in the community.

She has been happily married for 26 years to Charles Henderson. They have three handsome sons and three precious grandchildren.

www.ingramcontent.com/pod-product-compliance
Lightning Source LLC
Chambersburg PA
CBHW071432130726
47997CB00006B/2048